# HAPPY IS
# THE NEW HEALTHY

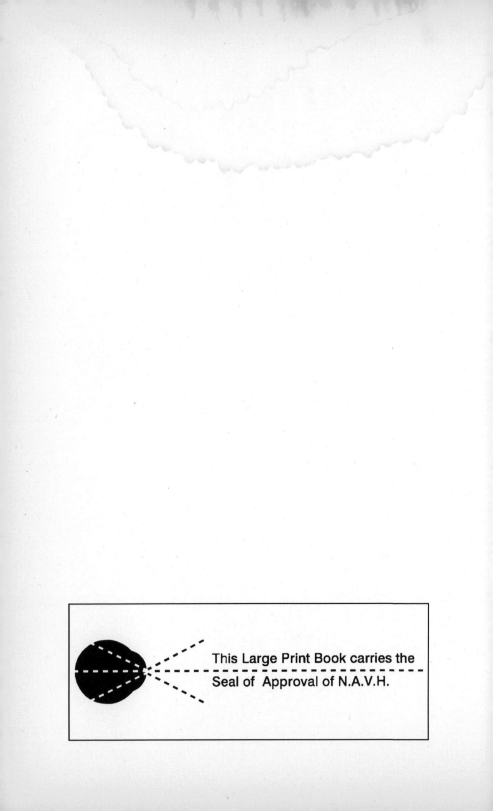

This Large Print Book carries the
Seal of Approval of N.A.V.H.

# HAPPY IS
# THE NEW HEALTHY

## 31 WAYS TO RELAX, LET GO, AND ENJOY LIFE NOW!

## DAVE ROMANELLI

**THORNDIKE PRESS**

*A part of Gale, Cengage Learning*

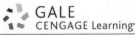
GALE
CENGAGE Learning·

Farmington Hills, Mich • San Francisco • New York • Waterville, Maine
Meriden, Conn • Mason, Ohio • Chicago

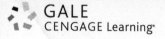
GALE
CENGAGE Learning®

Copyright © 2014 by David Romanelli.
Thorndike Press, a part of Gale, Cengage Learning.

LIBRARY OF CONGRESS CATALOGING-IN-PUBLICATION DATA

Romanelli, David.
    Happy is the new healthy : 31 ways to relax, let go, and enjoy life now! /
by Dave Romanelli. — Large Print edition.
    pages cm. — (Thorndike Press Large Print lifestyles)
    ISBN 978-1-4104-8366-9 (hardcover) — ISBN 1-4104-8366-5 (hardcover)
    1. Happiness. 2. Relaxation. 3. Health. 4. Large type books. I. Title.
BF575.H27R665 2015
158—dc23                                                        2015024146

Published in 2015 by arrangement with Skyhorse Publishing, Inc.

Printed in Mexico
1 2 3 4 5 6 7 19 18 17 16 15

To McKenna, my wife,
for your love and patience.

"Forget mistakes, forget failures, forget everything, except what you're going to do now and do it. Today is your lucky day."

— Will Durant,
Pulitzer Prize-winning author

# CONTENTS

# ACKNOWLEDGMENTS

My deepest thanks to Tony Lyons, Cat Kovach, and Jenn McCartney, from Skyhorse Publishing.

Thanks to everyone who has attended my events, retreats, and classes over the past fifteen years.

There are no words to express the gratitude I feel for my wife. Thank you for your loyalty, intuition, attention to detail, and risotto! I love you.

To my brother, for busting through boundaries and taking creativity to new heights.

Thanks to my family and friends for your love, support, and understanding of my circuitous path through life.

To everyone at Search and Care, for dedicating your lives to helping people age with grace.

Lastly, to the woman who inspired this book and passed away in June of 2014, a few days after her 111th birthday. In dedication to your undying spirit, may we all celebrate life, not tomorrow, but NOW!

# INTRODUCTION

They know the secret to life. Literally.

They are extremely rare, making up .00000085 percent of the global population. That means of the seven billion people on the planet, there are approximately sixty of these people alive today.

They are fueled by their resilience, humor, and joie de vivre.

They are extremely hard to find, and should you have the good fortune to spend a moment with one, embrace him or her with all your heart. Their wisdom will infect you.

They are scattered across the globe in third floor walk-ups of urban skyscrapers and in hidden, remote, off-the-grid villages.

They are supercentenarians, people who are 110 years or older. Supercentenarians are the most interesting people in the world.

After my last surviving grandparent passed

away in 2010, I saw the pain of growing old in America. My Grandma was always surrounded by loving relatives, but let's face it, as much as we love our parents and grandparents, they are not easily integrated into American culture.

Some have a room at an old age home. Yet such "retirement communities" or "assisted living residences" are symbolic of the value that we place on wisdom, something to look to on occasion, on holidays, maybe on Sundays, but certainly not a main influence in the American experience.

Think of the mistakes that could be avoided and the pain that could be alleviated with a little advice from a parent or grandparent. All too often, we ignore this advice, whether because we are stubborn, "independent," or disrespectful. It makes no sense.

For hundreds of years, people have mended broken hearts, endured tough times, and made difficult decisions. The solutions, potions, and remedies exist as richly in the minds and hearts of our elders as they do on internet search engines.

On the flip side, how frustrating to be in your senior years and have a lifetime of wisdom only to be perceived as an old body with an outdated perspective.

As Oscar Wilde famously said, "Youth is wasted on the young."

This misalignment of age and wisdom extends beyond the individual. Compared to the Asian and European nations, America is a very young country. If France is an old man, America is a scrappy youth exhibiting all the behaviors of a typical teenager. Moody, lots of ups and downs, physically strong, good at sports, likes to fight, and fights well. We are hormonal, beautiful, spunky, and we have lots of blemishes, like strip malls, rotting suburbs, and schools in disarray. Like many teenagers, Americans have little patience for wise advice from elders.

But there is hope. America is getting older. More people are embracing ancient traditions like yoga, meditation, and alternative medicine. And with such traditions come profound results. The twenty million Americans who practice yoga are more likely to breathe through stress. And the ten million Americans who meditate know the gift of mindfulness.

I have dedicated the past ten years to spreading the gospel to slow down, live in the moment, and celebrate life. I have traveled all over the country from my home in New York City to cities big and small, east and west. From Anchorage to Dallas, Los Angeles to Fayetteville, I have taught workshops and given speeches on embracing everyday passions as gateways to the present.

If there is one common gripe I hear from people, it is this: "How do I find more meaning in life? How do I live a life of passion and make a difference in this world? I don't have a second of free time in my day for my kids or my partner, let alone for meaning."

It's no mystery why meaning takes a back seat in our culture. We have giant financial burdens to meet each month in order to pay tuition, bills, mortgages, electricity, and to simply put food on the table. So we have no choice but to work hard at jobs that are often the farthest thing from our passions. Every moment of our day is consumed with emails, meetings, obligations, errands, text messages, and social media.

This is what makes supercentenarians so profoundly interesting. They provide a model of hope because they have endured the tough times, they have struggled through bad marriages, they have seen peace and war and peace and war. But through it all, they have refused to fall into the cracks of life and sputter into old age. What is their overarching secret?

French Renaissance writer Michel de Montaigne said, "The most evident token and apparent sign of true wisdom is a constant and unrestrained rejoicing."

In simpler words, the short cut, the secret, the means to meaning is CELEBRATION. As one of my buddies always says, "Find a little vacation every day!" Whether that means cranking the volume on Bob Marley's Three Little Birds (raises the vibration), or stepping away from the computer and savoring every sip of your morning coffee (slower is always better), or getting some sunshine on your face in the middle of a busy day (Vitamin D heals), these actions take a matter of seconds.

That is the essence of this book: the art of rising up and embracing all that is good in your life.

Of course, that sounds nice, but if you are not in a good state of mind, even Bob Marley cannot get through. For many, finding a little Zen, let alone reason to celebrate, is a tall order. Our brains are hard-wired with a negativity bias. According to neuropsychologist Rick Hanson, your brain is like Velcro for negative experiences and Teflon for positive ones. For most of human history, we were chased by predators or endangered by natural forces. So we are genetically wired to focus on what is wrong, what we do not have, what lurks in the unknown.

It takes practice to create a positivity bias, to be grateful for all you do have instead of all you do not have, all that is right instead of all that is wrong, all that feels good instead of all that aches.

In the pages to come, I will share ideas, inspirations, and meditations that will tilt your perspective toward the positive and give you damn good reason to celebrate your life!

But before you hear advice from a forty-year-old, better to hear it straight from someone who was born before JFK, before World War I, before Oklahoma, New Mexico, Arizona, Hawaii, and Alaska became states in the Union.

Let me tell you a little story about a supercentenarian named Katherine.

When my grandma passed away, I found a charity in New York City that helps the elderly who lack access to an old age home, money, family, or friends. Upon writing this book, their oldest client, a woman named Katherine, was 111 years old, or rather, 111 years young!

As I followed a social worker up the steps leading to Katherine's third story Upper East Side apartment, I wondered what it would be like to meet a woman who, upon turning eighty, had another lifetime (thirty-plus years) ahead of her. Would she be wired differently? Would there be something unique about her attitude, her energy, her eyes, her smile?

I walked through her front door and Katherine excitedly threw her arms in the air as if I was a long lost friend. While most elderly folks might fear the appearance of a new person in their home, Katherine was inherently trusting. As the quote goes, "Trust your journey." That was Katherine's mantra throughout her winding and weaving life. Born in South Dakota before it became a state, Katherine had a radio talk show, and she moved to New York City because she wanted the big city experience. She was married five times. A normal person might quit after the third or fourth marriage, but Katherine kept on truckin'!

While there were definite signs her body was starting to disconnect from her soul (including loose dentures that made it hard to understand her), Katherine had the vibrancy of a young child. Squirming around, flirting, a glimmer in her eyes, a passion to meet, to share, to taste . . . she was squeezing every possible ounce out of a life that began way back in 1903.

When the social worker put his hands on her asking, "Do you want to lie down?" she retorted, "Are you propositioning me?"

Ha! She was still as frisky as a teenager. Seriously, there were sparks flying off this woman, horsepower, an energy that said, "I am greater than my problems and stronger than my circumstances."

Here are Katherine's three tips to living a long and healthy life:

1. Sex
2. Vodka
3. Spicy food

This free-spirited, indulgent approach is best referred to as joie de vivre or "joy of life," one of the most common qualities shared by supercentenarians.

Claude Choules, the last surviving World War I veteran, passed away in 2011 at 110. He went swimming in the ocean every day until he was 100.

The oldest human of all time, Jeanne Calment, died in 1997 at 122 years young. Every week of her life, she ate two pounds of chocolate!

As I write this, Misao Okawa is the oldest person in the world. She attributes sushi and sleep to her 116 years of age.

And 115 year old Jerelean Talley is the third oldest person in the world at the moment I put these words to the page. She bowled until she was 104.

These might be some of the oldest humans ever to walk the earth, but they are the embodiment of a young and increasingly popular definition of wellness. They show us that real, lasting health is rooted in something deeper than the physical body.

They are living proof that aging gracefully is as much an attitude as it is genetics, diet, or exercise.

To anyone who could use a spark from Katherine's fire, Jeanne's joie de vivre, and Jerelean's vitality, I invite you to take a little journey. In the pages to come, I will lead you into a seventy million year old canyon, across frenetic streets in New York City, and through raging hurricanes in the Yucatan Peninsula. These stories will awaken you to a choice you make day by day and moment by moment: to wither with age, or to celebrate life!

My expertise lies at the intersection of modern and ancient. I take practices like yoga and meditation and infuse them with passion and pop culture. My Yoga + Chocolate, Yoga + Wine, and Yoga for Foodies experiences guide you into a relaxed state more conducive to savoring the simple pleasures.

What better than a slow sip of Cabernet, the sweet taste of exotic chocolate, and the scent of lavender from the French Alps to create a foundation of peace?

While presenting these yoga fusion experiences, I have conversed with thousands of Americans. Many have expressed the desire to be "well" but feel increasingly disconnected from the type of wellness we see on social media or strewn across glossy magazines. They say things like:

"I like yoga but just don't care about doing all these fancy yoga poses."

"I want to be healthy but not badly enough to drink green juice. I can't stand the taste of it. How do people drink that stuff?"

"I have no time in my day for anything but work and kids. How can I possibly get healthy when I barely have a free second to go to the bathroom? And who can afford those $100 yoga pants?"

The driving force behind this book is to make wellness more real and more relevant.

I will share very concrete ways to create the foundation for healthy living and a deeply fulfilling life without having to make crazy financial or physical sacrifices.

After a decade of touring and teaching, I have arrived at three guiding principles for life. These principles have nothing to do with far-fetched diets or expensive workout regimens. Rather, these principles inspire a state of mind, and a quality of heart amidst the realities we face every day: work, parenting, paying bills, insomnia, anxiety, stress, fear.

These are my three guiding principles:

## 1. Now Is Always the Best Moment!

We spend our lives waiting for something to happen that will give us permission to be well and happy. We are waiting to fall in love, waiting to find a better job, waiting to lose weight, waiting to get our certification, waiting to get a promotion, waiting to redo the kitchen, waiting to move into a new home, waiting, waiting, waiting. Waiting is a state of mind that never ends until that moment when you realize NOW is the best moment! That does not have to mean that NOW is the happiest moment, but it is always the moment you are most alive.

The following chapters share stories and simple tips on what you can do to celebrate life right this second.

From lessons learned amidst the raging rapids of a river rafting trip in Alaska to the titillating risk in my younger years of makin' the moves on the tenth grade beauty queen with whom I had .000001 percent chance, I have learned that life is not real unless it is happening NOW. That is why this is not a self-help book. This is a bust-loose book!

You do not want to end up in a hospital bed at the end of your life saying, "I wish, I regret, I should have, I could have."

And there's only one way and one word to change that attitude: NOW.

## 2. WELLNESS IS A STATE OF MIND.

I was recently driving through Los Angeles while visiting my parents for the year-end holidays. I saw countless fitness studios, tanning beds, beauty salons, personal trainer ads, health clubs, and juice bars. We go to great lengths for our bodies; what do we do for our minds? Where are the mental fitness studios and mind salons? Where are the personal trainers for the brain? A balanced state cleanses and strengthens the body and the mind.

If you are looking to be happier, to fulfill

your potential, to gain a competitive advantage, to heal mental health issues, herein lies the power of . . .

Wait. Before I say the word that has been associated with the worst kind of boredom, let me just say "it" is like easing your mind into a hot tub on a cold night. "It" is like the most loving hands massaging your mind after a stressful day. "It" is . . . meditation.

Meditation aids sleep, improves immune response, lowers blood pressure, alleviates stress and anxiety, boosts concentration, enhances pain response, lightens depression, the list goes on. And here is a little known secret: Once you find your meditation groove, it is like a trip to your Inner Hawaii. I equate the feeling of meditation with eating gnocchi on a black sand beach while getting a foot rub and watching the sunset.

Yet, so many say, "I want to try meditation, in the future. But not today. It's too slow for me."

Why is something with so many benefits . . . so difficult to embrace?

Your brain is the most complex object ever discovered in the universe. If you took a piece of your brain no bigger than the tip of a pen and stretched out all the neurons, they would extend two miles in length. That is how intricate the circuitry is in your brain. Yet with all that power, the average human has a loss of attention six to eight times per minute. With all our know-how, all our technology, all our expertise, we do not know how to harness our own brains.

In the pages to come, I am going to make meditation fun, and something that you will actually look forward to.

At the end of each of the following chapters, you will see the words "Meditate and Celebrate" followed by a thought to hold in your mind throughout the day. This is the first step in a meditation practice. Even before you sit still and close your eyes, just repeat the centering thought.

Most of us silently repeat negative thoughts to ourselves all day long. We say things like, "I don't have enough" or "I am overweight" or "I'm so stressed." It's no wonder we get stuck and frustrated.

Positive thinking works wonders on the mind. Try repeating "I am happy, I am awesome" one hundred times, and watch your mood instantly lighten.

### 3. HAPPY IS THE NEW HEALTHY.
Psychologist Ed Diener released a study showing that happiness is based on frequency of positive experience, not

intensity of positive experience. Instead of saving all your joy for that triple chocolate cupcake after work, the science shows that you will be happier spreading happiness throughout your day.

A pumpkin spice latte at breakfast, a walk in the sunshine after lunch, some exotic chocolate mid-afternoon, and a little jazz to wind down before heading home to catch a glimpse of that gorgeous crescent moon. None of these takes more than a few minutes, yet stacked together; they can turn an otherwise ordinary day into one for the ages.

Sounds easy enough.

Yet how often do you put your head on the pillow at night and not remember a single moment from your day? Do you have enough time to spend with your children, to enjoy nature, to listen to music, to read a book? Do you feel like your life is slipping through your fingertips? Am I asking too many questions?

In college, I asked so many questions that my friends stopped trying to answer and instead would say "Yeah Dave." I hope that spirit brings the following pages to life. I hope you think of me less as some preachy self-help author and more as your college buddy leading you on a road trip. You might ask, "Where are we going?"

We are going to bars, beaches, hair salons, and bar mitzvah dance floors all across the world.

Along the way, I will try my best to keep the questions to a minimum, but before we begin, can I just ask you one, well, maybe two questions?

Are you ready to celebrate? If not now, then when?

# 1
## Stick Your Paddle In

**Don't Feed the ~~Bears~~ Fears!**
My meditation space includes a stack of my favorite books, including Wayne Dyer's interpretation of the *Tao Te Ching,* Lawrence Kushner's *Honey from the Rock,* Joseph Campbell's *The Power of Myth,* some Frankincense oil (soothes the soul), and sage from Sedona, Arizona (clears the energy).

But the centerpiece of my meditation space is a giant statue of Shiva. A Hindu god who is often depicted dancing, Shiva embodies the constant flow of life and death, endings and beginnings. Shiva's energy infuses you with the vitality to deal with life's volatility.

And here's the thing. Vitality cannot be acquired or bought, learned, or inherited. Vitality is generated by uttering a simple word: YES!

As Rick Hanson writes in *Just One Thing,*

"The script is always changing, and saying 'yes' keeps you in the flow, pulls for creativity, and makes it more fun. Try saying 'no' out loud or in your mind. How's that feel? Then say 'yes.' Which feels better, opens your heart more, and draws you into the world?"

Whether you are out of shape, reeling from an injury, burdened by work, or crushed by love, the tendency is to turn away, to avoid change, to let the unruly brain make unhealthy decisions.

Sometimes we could all use that empowering reminder: "Turn around, dig deep, and say YES!"

I got my such reminder in the summer of 2008 on an adventure with my brother to Alaska.

Halfway down the river on a white water rafting trip, the guide tells us, "OK, this is the end of the trip for most of you. The rest of the river is Class 5, which means that this is very advanced. Great meeting you today."

The guide assumed we were a bunch of fancy pants yuppies from L.A., and we would not continue.

He was right.

I was gathering my stuff to exit the raft when my brother says, "You're not going anywhere! We didn't come all the way to Alaska to wuss out."

The rapids were so "gnarly" that the guide made us jump in the river to prepare for the pain of thirty-three degree water.

Mind you, the river was lined with bears searching for salmon, not to mention Class 5 super-intense rapids.

The guide gave us one piece of advice before starting.

"When you come to Alaska, you're gonna hear 'Don't feed the bears.' But I'm gonna tell you, 'Don't feed the fears!' " He continued, "If you cower in the raft, you're going to get sucked in. So engage, dig your paddle deep into the rapids. That's how you're going to stay in the raft."

My brother looked at me as if to say, "We didn't come to Alaska to pet each other and hold hands."

I would have been fine looking at some mountains, smelling the fresh air, maybe catching a fish or two. But bears? Freezing water? Rapids? I needed to be held.

We pushed off and down we went! The icy water felt like a million needles penetrating my skin. The force of the rapids converged on me like a 300 pound lineman. The screams of those in the raft reminded me of those heard in a death-defying drop on a massive roller coaster. This was quite possibly the most exhilarating adventure of my lifetime, partly because I moved through my fear, but mostly because of how I moved through it: fully engaged.

The rapids hit hard and bit hard. In a moment when I normally would have taken cover, instead I dug deep. Each intense stroke of the paddle into the freezing water was yet another way of saying that life-affirming word. YES!

## MEDITATE AND CELEBRATE

Stick your paddle in! Whatever you are facing right now, embrace it fully.

Easier said than done, right? As much as we hope for eternal serenity and utterly peaceful living, the universe is volatile and will challenge you in love, health, business, and faith.

What is currently stirring you up? Is it a move to a new home or city, changing jobs or maybe having a hard time finding one?

What are you fearing? Could it be a big presentation, job security, an upcoming social event, or love gone bad?

In what way do you feel overwhelmed? Maybe it is too much work, unceasing financial burdens, or overbearing responsibilities at home?

We all have something we are going through each and every day. You can shy away and hide, hoping to avoid the worst case scenario. Or you can stick your paddle in!

Engage.

One of my blog readers recently shared a story with me about engaging life when life demanded nothing less!.

Mary was supposed to get married on the auspicious date of 10-11-12. Everything was set to take place in Las Vegas. As she explained, "I was so excited I could burst."

Then on August 21, a day before their eight year anniversary together and less than eight weeks before the wedding, her fiancé backed out. He said, "There's a void in my life and I'm not happy."

Mary was devastated, to say the least.

On that date, 10-11-12, she still went to Vegas . . . with twenty-eight of her friends and family. The first night, she saw Vegas' famous long zipline, looked at her cousin, and said, "Fuck it! I'm going."

"I took a deep breath and told myself that this was the start of a new life, and I might as well step into it with bravery!"

Mary's one minute roaring down the zipline was her way of embracing the heartbreak, rather than avoiding it.

As the Alaskan guide screamed to us with the freezing water rushing into our eyes, "ROW, ROW, ROW!"

Or better yet, as Mary so fiercely shouted racing down that zip line: "YES! YES! YES!"

**When you find yourself hiding, ducking, running, you are "seeking freedom *from* life." Summon the vitality to look the other way and move toward your hopes and dreams. Repeat these words by Indian mystic Osho:**

*I seek freedom for life.*

*I seek freedom for life.*

*I seek freedom for life.*

# 2
## OVERCOME A CATEGORY 5 HURRICANE

**IN A TENSE SITUATION, RAISE YOUR VIBRATION!**

Remember Adam Sandler's "The Chanukah Song"? Here's a recap of the lyrics:

"When you feel like the only kid in town without a Christmas tree, here's a list of people who are Jewish, just like you and me."

On that note, I think it's time for "The Yoga Song" because, whether you love it or despise it, you cannot deny that the ancient practice of yoga is officially everywhere. Like religious brethren, yogis tend to feel a kindred connection with their fellow down doggers. So I came up with this little jingle:

There's Madonna toned and lean
Even Lebron's a yoga machine.

Jessica Biel and Gwyneth Paltrow
Shaquille O'Neal can do the crow

Jennifer Aniston in downward dog
Is that Jenny McCarthy in the frog?

They'll tell you in *People* and *Vanity Fair*
"Yoga's the answer, trust me, I swear!

"No need for therapy, I got a guru
Changed my physique, asked me out too
  (WHOOPS)."

CHORUS: Yoga, yoga, yoga, I think I can
Get an om tattoo, and a killer tan.
Then stretch on the beach, take a pic,
Hashtag "#NoEgo", but look at this trick!

Yoga is everywhere. If you don't do it, your kids do, or your partner, or your dentist, not to mention your favorite rock star, sports hero, and reality show host. Twenty million Americans get their stretch on.

But is the yoga really working?

Maybe you know that person with an awesome yoga practice, who has taken 800 hours of yoga training, who owns the best yoga mat and the most beautiful yoga clothes. And then you see this person on a plane or in a department store or in a parking lot . . . freakin' the hell out!

We all do it. Whether locking our keys in the car or getting a flat tire, the little things can cause major outbursts. These are the situations that reveal one's true character. It is easy to breathe and stay calm in a comfortable environment at your local yoga studio. But when you are faced with real life stressors, who do you become?

Wayne Dyer once said, "When you squeeze an orange, you get orange juice. When you squeeze a person, you never know what you're gonna get."

In September 2005, I led thirty-three people on a yoga retreat to Tulum, Mexico.

On the penultimate night of this glorious retreat, we went to sleep with vague knowledge of a very mild Category 1 hurricane several hundred miles off the coast. Nobody cared. We spent that night sitting around a campfire on the beach, hanging out, and livin' the moment!

Twelve hours later, I woke up to pandemonium. Overnight, that little hurricane underwent "extreme intensification" and jumped four categories to become Hurricane Wilma, a Category 5 monster with 175 miles per hour sustained winds.

You could see the sudden and dramatic shift. The skies darkened, the frothy surf whipped onto the once tranquil beach, the wind slapped the palm trees sideways. In the tropics, hurricanes can form suddenly, offering little time to react.

The teary-eyed manager of the very rustic retreat center at which we were staying had no evacuation plan.

There we were, in a very remote part of Mexico, with a Category 5 monster bearing down on us. It was hard to get a taxi to Señor Frogs on a lazy Wednesday, let alone arrange the evacuation of thirty-three very nervous human beings.

The next few hours exposed so much about the human character.

Many of those on the retreat were type A personalities, business owners or executives, with all their ducks in a row and plenty of money in the bank. But under pressure, they became rude, unruly, impossible.

"Dave, just make a decision already!"

"Look at you; you're just sitting there doing nothing. We're gonna die here if we don't figure this out NOW!"

"I never should have come on this retreat."

And yet, there was hope. Others on the retreat who had struck me as being a little kooky and dreamy (or possibly crazy) remained calm, cool, and collected. Many of these folks rose to the occasion. One helped find us transportation to the neighboring city of Mérida. Another called the airlines to change our flights. And yet another attempted to tell jokes and lighten the mood.

In her book *Unthinkable: Who Survives When Disaster Strikes,* Amanda Ripley describes "the disaster personality." Everyone reacts differently when they get squeezed. Some are heroic and calm, others get stressed and freak out, and some just freeze.

On September 28, 1994, the ferry SV Estonia sank in the Baltic Sea. One of the lucky survivors, Kent Härstedt, remembers the imperiled ship suddenly lurching thirty degrees before sinking. He fought his way to the ship deck expecting total chaos and panic. Much to his surprise, he saw passengers frozen, smoking cigarettes, as if nothing was happening. A few moments later, the ship sank upside down into the sea. Only 187 of the 989 people aboard the ship survived.

How could people just freeze in such a horrific scenario with their lives on the line?

In a more ancient and primitive habitat, humans were commonly endangered by wild animals, hunters, and the elements. They were accustomed to fight-or-flight scenarios and the subsequent rush of adrenaline that made them faster and stronger.

But in the modern day, when working in an office or driving in a car, we rarely face critical moments requiring important decisions with life-or-death consequences. If you are totally unfamiliar with the fight-or-flight feeling, adrenaline can be a destructive shock to your system.

Therein lies the importance of yoga and other mind-body practices. In a safe and protected environment, they induce heightened emotions and intense sensations. You practice "breathing through" rather than "reacting to" the intensity.

So what does it really mean to be a yogi? For those of us who cannot touch our toes or bust out the crazy yoga postures but still feel that we "get it," here is the true test:

When you are squeezed, stressed, and on the verge of freaking out, can you stay calm?

Joseph Campbell writes, "Opportunities to find deeper powers within ourselves come when life seems most challenging."

## MEDITATE AND CELEBRATE

Make an awesome choice.

Try this exercise. Hold your arms out to the sides of your body as if to form the letter T. Maintain this position for one to three minutes. At first this will seem easy, and you will be saying, "C'mon Dave." But then your shoulders will start to burn. As the burning increases in intensity, compare it to what you feel when rushing to the airport to catch your flight or overcome with too many emails and not enough time.

Breathe deeply, slow the mental process, and make the awesome choice to relax into the sensation rather than react to it.

Hopefully, you never have to face a serious crisis in your lifetime. But if you do, your behavior in a crisis says much about your character. The revelation is not to overcome crisis or outsmart it, but to know who you become in its midst.

**Next time you are squeezed and stressed, repeat:**

*Calm is the balm.*

*Calm is the balm.*

*Calm is the balm.*

# 3
# FREAKIN' GO FOR IT!

## SELF-DOUBT IS
## SELF-IMPRISONMENT

If you have ever been down on yourself, you know the feeling. You fall prey to the illusion that you can only get a certain kind of job, only earn a certain amount of money, only lose a certain amount of weight, only attract a certain kind of person (if anyone at all).

And then, one day (maybe today), you decide it's time for change. You are going to rip open the satchel containing your so-called "potential" and allow it to explode all over like a hot, glorious mess! You are going to embrace your inalienable right to beauty, abundance, health, and freedom.

This moment of liberation is usually a symbolic move, something that stands out in your timeline, your own version of Martin Luther King Jr's "I Have a Dream" speech.

We free ourselves in different ways at different stages in our lives, like moving on from a dark relationship or busting through an addiction.

Freedom is more than just one moment or one example. It is a daily affirmation, an ongoing process.

We face opportunities every day to grow, bloom, bust loose.

When those opportunities present themselves, we make a choice: fade into the shadows or step into the light.

In ninth grade, I decided to start lifting weights. If I could cultivate some biceps, maybe it would balance out the pimples on my face and enhance my appeal to the opposite sex.

So I joined the Nautilus Plus gym in the Town & Country mall in Encino, California. Not bothering to get a trainer, I'd show up and do curls with the barbells. That's all I'd do. Just curls. Oh yeah, I'd also stare at the prettiest girl I had ever seen, Andrea, a lovely blond in tenth grade at Birmingham High School in Tarzana.

I'd go to the gym almost every day and do curls while staring at Andrea on the stationary bike, Andrea on the Nautilus machine, Andrea talking to the trainer, Andrea breathing, smiling, existing.

My mom, with her thick New York accent, would drive me to Nautilus Plus and ask, "Don't you think working out every day is a little much?"

"I know, but look at this, Mom," and I'd flex my biceps.

"Maybe you should try for a little balance. Your dad said he'd pay for a trainer. You can't just have big biceps. It looks stupid."

"Big guns are where it's at," I'd say and again flex and stare at my emerging muscles. "The ladies love big guns."

"What ladies? Do you have a girlfriend?"

God I hated that question.

"Do you? Is there a special lady in your life?"

I'd slam the door and walk into the gym while feeling the ever-firmer tone of my biceps.

Flashing my membership card on one particular afternoon in March 1988, I saw something that I will never forget. Andrea was alone on the stationary bike. There were two rows of twenty bikes and each and every single bike was empty except for the one that Andrea was riding.

Oh my God, I thought. Could I actually talk to her? There she was with her perfect tan and long California blonde hair. And here I was, freckle on the lip, braces on the teeth, too much hair spray in the 'do, pimples spread like chocolate chips around my face, chicken legs, and big biceps.

With each step I took toward that stationary bike, I felt like I had ten pounds of weight in my shoes. Mind you, there were thirty-nine bikes available and I chose the one tucked into the far corner right next to her. A-w-k-w-a-r-d?

I can only imagine Andrea's inner dialogue, "I wonder if Billy likes me. What am I gonna wear to prom? These tights are uncomfortable. Who's this dork that just sat down next to me?"

I started peddling on the stationary bike while watching the time. Three minutes elapsed. I promised myself I would say something at three and a half. But I could not spit out a sentence. Four minutes passed. I promised I would say something at four and a half. But I was at a loss for words.

Finally, five minutes after the extreme weirdness of sitting on the bike right next to Andrea, I spit out, "Y'know why he's called Magic Johnson, right?"

I could not think of anything else to say.

"Um, not really sure. Cause he's good at basketball?" she hesitantly answered.

"Well that, but also cause, his ah, Johnson,

is Magic."

"How do you know that?" she asked, smirking.

"I read it in *Mad Magazine.*"

It was Revenge of the Nerds at Nautilus Plus.

We chitchatted for what must have been twenty minutes. She gave me her number before leaving to go home. To make a long story short, we had some fantastic phone conversations until she suddenly stopped talking to me a few months later. It turns out one of my friends sold me down the river and told Andrea all about my huge crush.

But I was forever transformed.

I realized, you never know unless you try. Søren Kierkegaard said, "To dare is to lose one's footing momentarily. To not dare is to lose oneself."

## MEDITATE AND CELEBRATE

Liberate yourself from self-doubt. Today is your day to freakin' go for it!

Everything is possible in a world of action.

If there is something you want, ask for it! How could someone possibly know what you need unless you ask?

If you are seeking to connect with

someone who seems out of your league, reach out and be tenacious. There are so many people with talent and so few with real tenacity.

If there is someone you want to ask out, but you fear being rejected, do it anyway. If the person is right, your soul will find a way past pretensions and into their heart. But you have to give your soul that chance.

So keep shooting, keep daring, and keep trying.

Civil rights leader Howard Thurman said, "Don't ask what the world needs. Ask what makes you come alive, and go do it. Because what the world needs is people who have come alive."

Step outside of your home, your fears, your comfort zone — and give life a chance.

Best-case scenario . . . MAGIC! Worst-case scenario . . . FREEDOM.

**When you are standing at the edge, wondering if you should take the leap, here is some extra encouragement:**

*Aim high, then let go. Relax, trust the flow.*

*Aim high, then let go. Relax, trust the flow.*

*Aim high, then let go. Relax, trust the flow.*

# 4
# CATCH A RIDE ON THE UPWARD SPIRAL

## IT TAKES A REAL BADASS TO BE TRULY GRATEFUL

Certain human abilities are very rare. Sometimes they are an emotional state, like sustained bliss. Do you know someone who is always happy? Other times it is an athletic skill, which of course leads to great fame and fortune. And even more rare is a unique mental capacity. My dad's friend is the fastest backward talker in the world, or, as he would say, "dlrow eht ni reklat drawkcab tsetsaf."

Here are some very rare skills, in no particular order or relevance:

### 5. Hitting a Baseball

Considering that a major-league pitch can reach speeds more than 95 mph, hitters have only 0.4 seconds to find the ball, decide where the ball is going, and swing the bat. At the time of printing, there were only twenty-two people on the planet able to .300 or over against major league pitchers. That's twenty-two out of seven billion.

## 4. Raising a Child

Upon writing these words, I have a baby on the way. So I cannot write from experience. But I have heard parenthood is amazing . . . and profoundly challenging. Everyone says raising children is both the hardest and best thing you will ever do.

## 3. Saving a Penalty Kick

On the soccer field, the goalkeeper's job is to protect a goal that is 24 feet wide and eight feet high — 192 square feet waiting to swallow a ball about 9 inches in diameter. During a penalty kick, the goalie has 0.25 seconds to move and block a ball traveling at more than 60 mph.

## 2. Maintaining a Healthy Marriage

I am only in year three but some of you going on twenty, thirty, and forty years will attest to the work required to sustain an enduring relationship. When you see a couple deeply in love after being together for thirty years, that is special, and rare.

# 1. Feeling Sudden Gratitude

In a culture that always pushes us to do more, earn more, and buy more, gratitude is elusive.

I recently heard about an executive who received his end-of-year bonus. It was eight figures! That means somewhere north of $10,000,000. And the executive was pissed. He felt he deserved more.

This executive clearly suffers from a mental disease called EINE – Enough Is Never Enough.

EINE can lead to incredible success, and an empty pit in the soul.

For instance, I was sick to my stomach when famed University of Alabama football coach Nick Saban said, after winning a National Championship, "We'll take a few days and start getting ready for next season."

Hey coach, what message does that convey? What about taking time to be thankful? We have to stop and celebrate life, every day, not to mention after winning a national championship. And that's why sudden gratitude is one of the hardest and rarest skills. When I say "sudden," I mean the ability to stop right now and say thank you for all that is good. Try it.

"Thank you for my life. 151,000 people

on the planet die each day. You just never know. While I'm here, I will enjoy it."

"Thank you for my comfort. Of the two billion children on the planet, one billion live in poverty. I have a roof over my head and that is a blessing."

"Thank you for the snack I am about to enjoy. I wish I could share it with every single one of the approximately one billion people on this planet who go to sleep hungry every night. I will savor each bite."

For some reason, gratitude does not come easily. Robert Emmons, author *The Psychology of Gratitude,* writes, "Gratitude is morally and intellectually demanding."

In other words, you have to be a badass to be grateful! It's easy to wake up in the morning and fixate on the mess of clothes strewn across the house, the dirty dishes in the kitchen, the impossibly long list of what needs to get done. It takes mental strength to shift your attention and see all that is well and all that is right.

Do not wait. This is not a message to practice tomorrow. If you are not grateful for what you have right now, how will you be grateful for what you hope to have in the future?

I recently discovered Uber, a mobile app

that connects passengers with drivers of vehicles-for-hire.

On a balmy late summer evening, an Uber driver pulled up to the curb. As I restlessly tried to open his trunk, he politely offered to help me with my luggage. I could tell he was a gentle soul. "Gentle souls" often have beautiful stories, and I wanted to learn more.

His name was Richard. He was a Pakistani immigrant who spent the past decade working for a limo company that cheated him out of fares. He squeaked by at near-poverty, spending day after day, grinding it out in New York City gridlock.

But Richard kept his heart open and met a wonderful woman. They married several years ago, yet he still described her with words like "magnificent," "special," "a dream come true." Hey, when 50 percent of marriages end in divorce, it is always wonderful to hear a man tell you how much he loves his wife.

Lesson 1: If you have love, especially self-love, you have fullness in your heart. That is the seed of health and wealth and all good things.

Richard then heard about Uber, quit his job, and started fresh. He became his own boss and set his own hours, as Uber drivers do. He was making three times as much income.

"The veil has been lifted," Richard proclaimed to me, as we slowly made our way through the traffic. "I don't know if it's God, or what, but I am blessed."

Lesson 2: Blessings accumulate.

By expressing deep gratitude for his beloved wife, Richard opened up to more good fortune. One blessing leads to the next much like an upward spiral builds momentum. To get sucked in and catch a ride, start at the bottom of the vortex. In other words, start by appreciating the little things.

If you are grateful for the little things, they become the big things.

If you are grateful for the big things, they become the magnificent things.

If you are grateful for the magnificent things, they become miraculous things.

As Richard dropped me off at home, I felt lighter, at ease. I sensed that the complex formula for happiness that I was seeking to understand could be reduced to two simple words.

Thank You.

Catch a ride on the upward spiral.

Take a moment to think of five things or people for whom you are grateful. Start small and it will not be long before you are feeling big.

1. Someone who loves you, like a partner, child, or friend.
2. The roof over your head that allows you to sleep comfortably.
3. The food in your kitchen that nourishes you.
4. The clothes in your closet that comfort you.
5. Your breath which grants the gift of life.

I once heard this particularly fitting analogy:

Imagine you bring an expensive bottle of wine to the host of a party. Days and weeks go by, and the host never takes the time to thank you. You would be much less likely to bring this host another really nice gift in the future.

The universe works the same way. If you fail to express gratitude for your blessings, why would the universe bestow more of them?

Express sudden gratitude. The busier your schedule, the darker your mood, the deeper your envy . . . the more powerful this practice becomes. Repeat:

*Thank you.*

*Thank you.*

*Thank you*

# 5
# LOSE A BAR MITZVAH LIMBO CONTEST

## BEGINNINGS REQUIRE ENDINGS

If the caterpillar doesn't create a cocoon, it doesn't become a butterfly. So it goes with the human experience. There are tests and trials we must pass in order to evolve. But because of our higher brain functions (aka fears, worries, neuroses), sometimes we choose to skip the cocoon process. And then we wonder why our wings never grow.

This cocoon process is often known as a rite of passage, a ritual or test that marks your passing from one stage of life to another, from a caterpillar to a butterfly.

Mythologist and writer Joseph Campbell describes how an Aboriginal boy is brought into the field and put through an ordeal involving circumcision, subincision, and drinking of men's blood. After this rite of passage, the boy is officially a man and as Campbell said, "There's no chance of relapsing into boyhood after that."

Are there any rites of passage remaining in modern day America? Those rare few that we do honor tend to become lavish parties and social affairs, masking their deeper meaning. For instance, in the Jewish religion, when children turn thirteen, they have a bar or bat mitzvah and become men and women, able to participate in all areas of Jewish community life. However, in the modern day, the bar mitzvah has become more about the party, the flash, the DJ. It's as if God stopped asking on this sacred day, "Are you ready to become a man or a woman?" and instead asked, "Can you throw a good party?"

In seventh grade my face looked like the dark side of the moon with craters, pocks, and its own oxygen-depleted atmosphere (or so it seemed if you saw the expression of one girl's face who I asked to go steady).

"Um, ah, um, ah . . . can I tell you next year?" she answered.

I was on the outside looking in, someone less than popular, you might say. I did not wear fashionable clothes, have slick hair, or date the cool girls. Well, to be honest, I did not date any girls, let alone the cool ones.

My mom had to recruit kids to come to my bar mitzvah. She was like a Jewish version of John Calipari, the college basketball coach who is known for his sly recruiting tactics.

There were four other bar mitzvahs on June 21, 1986, so my mom had to call other kids' moms and do some clever maneuvering to make sure their kids picked my bar mitzvah over others.

The big day came and I had five friends show up including my crush, Kate, and her posse. My mom came through big.

Everyone danced to the hits from 1986 including "Broken Wings" by Mr. Mister, "How Will I Know" by Whitney Houston, and "You Give Love a Bad Name (Shot Through The Heart!)" by Bon Jovi. The guests had their picture taken in front of a *Sports Illustrated* magazine backdrop. Everything was perfect.

But due to the lack of competition at the party, I was in a final showdown with my friend Lance during the limbo contest. Lance let me win, and that was embarrassing. Nobody wants to beat the bar mitzvah boy. That is like dunking on a five-year-old in a game of Nerf basketball.

In case you are not familiar with limbo, the objective is to duck under a pole, which gets lower and lower each round. Limbo is for boys, not men. Men are supposed to get bigger and bigger, not smaller and smaller.

All these years, I have had a part of me that still feels like a boy, ducking below life's challenges just like I ducked below the limbo stick at my bar mitzvah.

Perhaps there is a test you have avoided, a rite of passage you have not completed?

Whether it is an ability to be alone and at peace (a wisdom acquired through introspection), or a proper appreciation for the value of a dollar (which comes from working hard), or being mindful of another's feelings (best learned when you are heartbroken and spend hard time in The Pain Chamber), all are best assimilated via a rite of passage, a defining moment that solidifies the message in your mind, body, and spirit.

Since my college days, I've had the nickname Yeah Dave.

I used to ask questions that didn't have answers, so my buddies stopped trying to answer and would instead say, "Yeah Dave."

It stuck around past college into my adulthood. I still like to ask questions.

At home, I'm allowed one such question per day. It's a tight quota or else I drive my wife crazy. But it's my way of stretching my mind (aka blowing a bubble in my head).

"What would you do if you were waiting

for your first date with a guy and he showed up with a huge moose knuckle (aka jacked his pants up above his waist)?"

"What would you do if I danced with my arms cranking back and forth like a freestyle swimmer and kept shouting 'Takarate!' every time I pretended to come up for air?"

"If you had to choose, would you rather have a really small nose and really big eyes, or really small eyes and a really big nose?"

I could go on and on and on.

Yes, this is a somewhat adolescent quality that can be fun the first time you meet me, and funny when channeled properly into my writing, but more often than not it became like a tooth that never fell out and blocked my other teeth from coming in.

We all have those character traits from our youth (e.g., competitiveness or silliness or drive) that are wild and crazy and must be properly harnessed in our later years. You might say my penchant for asking questions was left unchecked.

On an otherwise ordinary summer night while riding in a New York City taxi with a college friend, I asked him one of my infamously random questions:

His response: "Yeah Dave, less questions, more answers!" BOOM, lightning struck!

Less questions. More answers. Less

insecurity. More self-esteem. Less worry. More faith.

We reach moments in our lives where it is very clearly the time to graduate, moments where we realize we have the knowledge we need to take the test, to turn the page, and evolve.

At forty years old, I realize there are as many people younger than me as there are older. And while questions are always good, and curiosity is a sign of intelligence, I realized that night in the taxi it was time to rise up and step over the limbo stick.

After so many years and so much experience, one best start answering questions . . . along with asking them.

## MEDITATE AND CELEBRATE

Close a chapter on your past that lingers in your present.

My bar mitzvah had always been a painful memory. I was so worried about having enough friends in attendance that I never really basked in the symbolism of the event.

So on this page right here, I declare my friend Lance, who finished second in the limbo contest, as the honorary champion. Congratulations, Lance. But more importantly, I am changing the way I see my bar mitzvah. It was an intimate celebration of life.

From today forward, I will tell a different story about my bar mitzvah. The band Leonard Neil jammed all the best eighties hits, the hairdos were mega (and flammable from the hairspray), and my braces glimmered in the dance floor spotlights!

What is a chapter in your life that could use a final sentence and a little closure?

Maybe it's an ex you are ready to forgive and forget, or possibly a decision you made, a person you rejected, a job you said no to and have spent way too much time regretting.

Your life is unfolding in front of you right this very second. Step up and step over whatever is holding you back.

**If you are clinging tightly to the past, remember this nugget of brilliance from author Richard Bach:**

*"The river delights to lift us free, if only we dare let go."*

*"The river delights to lift us free, if only we dare let go."*

*"The river delights to lift us free, if only we dare let go."*

# 6

## CURE YOUR FEAR

**F.E.A.R — FORGET EVERYTHING
AND ~~RUN~~ RISE**

Father's Office is a small restaurant and bar on Montana Avenue in Santa Monica, California, that features the most amazing burger I have ever had. Vegetarians, close your eyes and hold your breath. Dry-aged sirloin topped with applewood-smoked bacon compote, maytag blue and gruyere cheeses, caramelized onions, and arugula on a freshly baked French roll. Along with a Chimay beer and sweet potato fries, the Father's Office burger is a wave of sensory pleasure that evokes a perpetual yet silent "yahooooooo!" as each bite builds upon the next.

One thing to note about Father's Office. You don't just show up, get a table, and place your order. There is always a line out the door. The rules may have changed, but when I frequented the place, after finally entering the front door, you would have to fight your way through the crowd to find a seat.

The bar was at least two rows deep and if you were lucky enough to find a table, you would be sitting with four strangers, some of whom had driven fifty miles to this legendary spot where art and pleasure meet the carnal craving for a juicy taste of red meat.

On one evening, I waited in line for thirty minutes before fighting my way to the bar, where one seat happened to open. Thanks to my being an experienced Father's Office veteran, I pounced on it with a quick first step. I ordered my delicious Chimay beer and waited with great excitement for the sweet potato fries and burger. My moment in burger heaven was just seconds away!

NOTE: I am a germ freak. I hate making contact with door knobs in public bathrooms, shaking hands with strangers, or holding on to the handrails when riding the New York City subway. So when I'm about to eat fries and a burger (let alone a Father's Office burger), I'm in total germ lockdown.

As I sat there waiting, anticipating, my wonderful friend Dawn and her date Brian wrestled their way to the bar. Dawn was a pleasant and cheery type who I was oh-so-happy to see. But then it happened. She introduced me to her date, who held out his hand to shake mine.

Oh my God, I thought. There was no way I could shake his hand.

Going to the bathroom to wash my hands would be a ten-minute obstacle course through the crowded bar, and surely I would lose my seat. At that moment, I looked down and saw my burger and fries had just arrived. I looked back at Brian's hand. I looked down at my burger and fries.

I made a decision and didn't shake his hand.

Later, Dawn explained in her sweet, polite vernacular, "When there's a perfectly nice person who wants to connect with you, and you choose dead meat over a loving heart, there's a problem."

She was right. In that moment, I chose fear over love.

Whether it is germs, rejection, or darkness, fear manifests in so many forms.

I walked around New York City with a film crew and interviewed people about their fears. The most common were fear of being alone (Monophobia), fear of commitment (Gamophobia), fear of failure (kakorrhaphiophobia), fear of poverty (Peniaphobia), fear of death (Necrophobia), fear of ladders (Stepnophobia), and fear of in-laws (Soceraphobia).

Here are a few others which you may relate to:

Venustraphobia — Fear of beautiful women
Pogonophobia — Fear of beards
Arachnophobia — Fear of spiders
Botanophobia — Fear of plants
And of course . . . Mysophobia — Fear of Germs

Why do such strange things provoke such intense reactions? Thousands of years ago, our ancestors were exposed to raw elements and wild animals. The slightest sound or movement would trigger a fight-or-flight response. The sudden boost of adrenaline enabled them to run faster and improve their chance of escape.

While we no longer are facing wild animals and raw elements, we have the same software in our brains which explains why the little things can trigger intense reactions.

We have the ability to override that ancient software. As Anais Nin said, "People living deeply have no fear.

Whatever you are afraid of — germs, rejection, darkness, failure — get under it and come from a deeper place.

Carl Hammerschlag is a medical doctor who spent many years living on American Indian reservations. His healing stories have a way of cutting through to precise and deep spots in our soul that are well beyond the reach of the scalpel.

Dr. Hammerschlag tells of the coastal Salish Native American tribe of the Pacific Northwest and their story of a double-headed snake monster named Sisquiutl. The snake monster is sixty feet long and as big as a giant redwood. At each end is a huge, swiveling head that enables it to see in every direction. Nothing falls outside its vision. If you come upon Sisquiutl, your instinctive reaction is to run. If it sees you move, Sisquiutl will come after you.

The Salish say the only way to escape the monster is to stand still. By standing still, Sisquiutl will approach you slowly, moving first one end, then the other, until it traps you between both its heads. Then suddenly it will see itself and, horrified by its own reflection, slither away.

This is the only way to overcome fear: not

with force or effort but with stillness and grace.

**The next time you feel fear getting the best of you — when you are dealing with your finances, boarding a plane, or facing a health issue — remember:**

**Fear stands for:**

*Forget Everything and Rise.*

*Forget Everything and Rise.*

*Forget Everything and Rise.*

# 7
# TAKE ONE MINUTE
## FOR LOVE

---

**"LOVE IS A WEAPON OF LIGHT."**
**Yehuda Berg**

Words are nice. But there is nothing like touch to express love.

So why do Americans have such a strange relationship with touch?

In the 1960's, pioneering psychologist Sidney Jourard studied the conversations of friends in various parts of the world as they sat together in cafés. His findings were astonishing, and remain relevant 50 years later.

— In the United States, in bursts of enthusiasm, the friends touched each other only two times on average.

— In France, the number shot up to one hundred and ten touches.

— In Puerto Rico, friends touched each other a whopping one hundred and eighty times in one hour!

If one hundred and eighty touches in one

hour is hard to fathom, you are not alone. Many of us will go days, weeks, even months without a loving touch. Has it been too long since you felt the warmth of massage or the healing connection of a loving embrace?

On a recent trip to India, I noticed a very common sight: two straight men holding hands. Whether walking home from a bar or on a leisurely lunchtime stroll, the men held hands simply to express their friendship.

It is not just in India. In many Arab nations, it is very normal for straight men to hold hands.

Said Musa Shteiwi, a sociology professor at the University of Jordan, "Arab culture has historically been segregated, so emotions and feelings are channeled to the same sex. Men spend a lot of time together, and these customs grew out of that."

Being that I am a touchy-feely wellness guy, I thought it was a nice custom and wondered why it was so taboo for straight men to hold hands in America. A short time after returning home from India, I was watching the Lakers basketball game with my friend Brock. We were having a great time watching a nail-biter of a game and screaming at the TV. The Lakers were in a tense time-out.

I thought this would be the perfect moment to hold Brock's hand and enjoy this awesome moment together. But Brock looked at me as if someone had just poured spicy sauce in his eyeballs. He was dismayed, to say the least. The rest of the evening was very awkward, and that was the first and last time I tried to hold a buddy's hand.

For the record, the most touchy-feely teams in the National Basketball Association are the most connected and most successful. A *New York Times* article published in 2010 stated, "Good teams tended to be touchier than bad ones. The most touch-bonded teams were the Boston Celtics and the Los Angeles Lakers, two of the league's top teams (in 2010); at the bottom were the mediocre Sacramento Kings and Charlotte Bobcats."

Why?

Touch releases oxytocin, a hormone that helps create a sensation of trust, and reduces levels of the stress hormone cortisol.

But it goes far beyond trust. Touch is at the very core of our well-being. In the early 1900's, 99% of babies in orphanages in the United States died before they turned seven months old. The babies did not die from malnourishment or infectious diseases. They died from a condition called "marasmus," caused by lack of touch.

As babies need touch to survive, adults need touch to thrive. Yet, we go far too long without a loving touch. According to Matthew Hertenstein, Director of the Touch and Emotion Lab at DePauw University, touch deprivation is a real thing. He said, "Most of us, whatever our relationship status, need more human contact than what we are getting."

This does not have to mean going to extremes and starting your own cuddle puddle. Instead, how about a gentle touch on the shoulder or occasionally holding another's hand, or if you really want to get crazy . . . a long, deep, loving hug?

As they say, a little love goes a long way.

## MEDITATE AND CELEBRATE

There are 1,440 minutes in a day. Can you take just one minute each day for love? Reach out and send someone an uplifting email. Surprise another with a cup of coffee. Uplift a friend or co-worker with a heartfelt compliment. Little surprises are few and far between in today's busy world. This is not rocket science. It is merely one minute in your day.

My personal preference is the one-minute hug.

I performed a social experiment and walked around New York City with a film crew to see if I could give the world's moodiest people a One-minute hug. Once you get past the tough exterior shell, New Yorkers are no different than every other human on earth. We all need more love.

After posting the one minute mug video online, I had a contest asking viewers to pass the video on to their friends to be entered in the One-Minute Hug Sweepstakes. I promised to show up at the winner's house to personally deliver a one-minute hug.

I received entries from all over the United States. Along with their entries, people shared stories about giving One-Minute hugs to family, co-workers, and friends.

One spin teacher in Phoenix wrote, "Today, I brought my class your message about the one-minute hug. I asked for volunteers to get off their spin bikes and hug for one minute. I am thrilled to tell you, I had people throwing up their hands with excitement, 'Pick me! Pick me!'

"As the class continued, we timed our one-minute hugs. Everyone was so happy, talking to one another, dancing while hugging. They made it look effortless! We do need more love in this world, so let the hugging begin!"

And if you are touch-adverse, how about a little science to push you over the edge and into another's arms. A University of North Carolina study showed that blood pressure was significantly lower in huggers versus non-huggers. In other words, hugs heal.

So whatever you are facing today, before you look to the medicine cabinet, open your arms. A hug might not cure your problem, but it will heal your soul. And that is always the best place to start.

**Next time you are facing a rift between you and your colleague, arguing with your partner, or griping at your children, save yourself a whole lot of time and trouble. Unleash your weapon of light.**

**Remember:**

*Love heals the soul.*

*Love heals the soul.*

*Love heals the soul.*

# 8
# GO WITH GRAY

**YOUTH IS AN ATTITUDE!**
There was a hush in the room, something that you might experience in the emergency room or possibly at a morgue. We studied one another with a look of mourning. There was great loss of hair, muscle tone, and vitality. Many came alone. All seemed to be forced awkwardly into this moment. One woman gazed at me with hollow eyes as if to say, "The end is near."

But we were not in a hospital ward or at an accident scene, and nobody had died.

It was a high school reunion. Have you been to one lately?

With the exception of a few folks, it seemed that most of my classmates were tending to the grueling demands of life. When we start to worry more than imagine, and to regret more than dream, we put the hand brakes on. We feel the friction against our skin and bones, and it hurts, it scrapes, it incinerates our vitality.

Or so I have learned.

I recently turned forty, at which time I was told by a friend, "Welcome to middle age." As seen at the high school reunion, most of my friends now have gray hairs, and it's never much of anything to let your guy friends know they are aging. But at this reunion, an old friend, Cheryl, was different. She had a vibrant energy and seemed to be embracing the aging process.

I said to her, "Heyyyyy, Cheryl, you look great! Better than anyone here. If it wasn't for your gray hair, I'd totally think you were still in your twenties!"

"Yeah Dave," she said angrily mocking my supposedly positive nickname.

I wandered off to chat with some of my former classmates. But nobody intrigued me like Cheryl. Her skin shined, her aura glowed, and her energy flowed. Her vibe was infectious.

I brought her a drink and said, "Cheryl, I really admire you, seriously, for going with gray. Most women would cover that up, and it's so cool how true you are to yourself!"

I really meant what I said. She stood out in the most wonderful way.

Evidently, forty-something year old women do not like to be told they have gray hair, especially by men.

She just looked at me, and I felt like Sookie Stackhouse from the TV show *True Blood.* Surely I could read her mind. I was certain she was thinking, "David Romanelli is a fuckface. Why did I come here?"

And then, amazingly, she actually said, "David Romanelli. You're a fuckface. Why did I come here?"

It goes without saying: aging is a very touchy subject.

When my wife pointed out the first grays in my beard, I looked twice, and then a third time, and then one more time to see if she was correct. And she was. The first glimmer of twilight, however distant it might be, had arrived in the form of four gray hairs in my beard. I did not expect it, at least not for another few years. I was mildly disappointed. But why?

We are so youth-obsessed in America that gray hair is perceived as a negative thing. In fact, 75 percent of American women and a growing percentage of American men color their hair. Look up "cover gray hair" on the Internet and you'll get hundreds of millions of results.

One place in the world where things are different (very different) is the Caucasus region of southern Russia in a place called

Abkhazia. As reported in John Robbins' book *Healthy at 100,* Abkhazia has an extraordinary number of people who are 100 years or older. Abkhazians are considered more beautiful in their old age than in their youth.

To tell an elder Abkhazian that she looks young is considered an insult. To tell the same person "You're looking old today" is a compliment.

Wrinkles are battle scars, the coolest of cool in the land of Abkhazia.

Can you imagine if I had said to Cheryl, "Not only do I love your gray hair, but your wrinkles are freakin' fabulous!"?

So here is the question. If you are going to great lengths to hide your wrinkles and gray hairs, is that really the authentic you?

Not to say changing your hair color is bad. But what is bad is getting down on yourself about a streak of gray, or a new crease on your face, or a little extra padding.

As Douglas MacArthur said, "Youth is not entirely a time of life — it is a state of mind. It is not wholly a matter of ripe cheeks, red lips, or supple knees. It is a temper of the will, a quality of the imagination, a vigor of the emotions."

Go with Gray.

In any way you are fighting the aging process, loosen your grip on the past and let the vitality of the present moment surge into your veins, spread across your skin, and revitalize your soul.

As I approached forty, I found myself focusing on all the things I had not yet accomplished, like starting a family and living in a certain house in a certain neighborhood. In other words, I was looking back at my regrets, a ripe condition for aging to strike hard and fast.

I received an email from a reader that I will never forget. Mary wrote, "I was having a little struggle with turning forty until I was told by my dying sister (cancer sucks), 'Oh babe, what I would do with another year. Please promise me that you will celebrate another year every day.' "

Celebrate Another Year Every Day.

On the eve of my fortieth birthday, I went to a cheap Mexican restaurant with great margaritas and wore a big ass sombrero. It was my way of saying, a year older and a year lighter!

The next day, I sent out a blog entitled "My 40th Birthday Bash." With such a subject, one might expect to open the blog and find images of a fancy party with a big birthday cake, flowing champagne, and the other aspirational desires and experiences we see on our social media newsfeed.

But if you opened the blog, it was just a picture of me in a big ass sombrero at a cheap Mexican restaurant blowing out a meager candle in a floppy slice of flan. And you know what? I had a blast!

The next day, another reader, Brian, reached out:

"I am turning 50, the BIG FIVE O, and I am really struggling with it. I have never struggled with any age before . . . so this is all unexplored territory. I feel like I have 'missed my mark' developmentally. I have the best job on the planet. I love all of my coworkers. I have a good home, a pet, my daughter is in graduate school. My life is fabulous, and yet, I feel I have failed. Your picture in the [big ass sombrero] made me step back and take a deep breath."

The truth be told, underneath that big ass sombrero, I had all those same thoughts . . . and yet I still had a blast.

If you are struggling with the aging process . . .

If you can't bear to look at pictures from your youth . . .

If you can't see past the color of your hair,

the shape of your body, or the condition of your skin . . .

Here's a thought to consider before your next high school reunion.

American actor John Barrymore said, "You don't age until your regrets outnumber your dreams."

**Instead of looking back at the blemishes of the past, rekindle the energy of the present. Repeat:**

*Presence is timeless beauty.*

*Presence is timeless beauty.*

*Presence is timeless beauty.*

# 9

# EMBRACE THE POWER OF 1:11

## THE PRESENT MOMENT IS ALWAYS ONE BREATH AWAY

At a bachelor party in Las Vegas, one of my college buddies pulled an old VHS tape out of his suitcase. We proceeded to watch a video of a fraternity party from our senior year in college. This video took us back to a time, 1995, when no one had an email address, let alone a cell phone. As if moving in slow motion, everyone in the video was doing something that rarely happens in today's world: looking at each other, listening to each other, living in the moment.

How things have changed!

Getting your first cell phone was a before-and-after moment. Before, there were spare minutes with which you could breathe, relax, converse. And of course, there were more inconveniences. How did we get in touch during the pre-cell phone era? Pay phones, answering machines, beepers?

82

Now, you can reach anyone instantly. And with this instant access comes a whole new set of issues. A revealing photo of your big night out can ruin your career. An angry email can blow up your relationship. And an auto-correct texting disaster can . . . well . . . um . . .

Let me explain.

It was late at night and I sat in bed, bleary-eyed, checking a few recent text messages.

One lady, Rainie, wrote, "I'm excited to see you tomorrow at your workshop. I'm bringing a whole bunch of my friends."

I replied via text, "Great, Rainie! Can't wait to see you and your posse."

I am convinced that the person who invented the "auto-correct" technology is a dirty old man. The phone changed the word "posse" to "pussy".

In other words, Rainie was about to read, "Great, Rainie! Can't wait to see you and your pussy."

Shoot! I looked at the clock; 11:52 PM. Was it too late to call her?

Ring, ring, ring.

"Hello?" she answered, sounding half-asleep.

"Rainie, hi! I'm so sorry to be calling this late. It's Dave Romanelli."

"Oh, hey." Long silence. Clearing her

throat, Rainie said, "Y'know I'm married, right?"

"Honey it's my yoga teacher," Rainie quickly told her grumpy husband in bed next to her.

I continued, "Listen, Rainie, I totally apologize. I just wanted to give you a heads-up that I tried to thank you for bringing your pussy, I mean posse, and my cell phone wrote pussy when I meant to say posse."

"What? Who in the world?" the suddenly heated husband grunted, having overheard me say pussy to his wife in the middle of the night.

"Rainie, is this the guy you were saying touches your thighs in down dog?"

"No, that's another guy; this is the chocolate guy," Rainie told her husband.

A few awkward moments later, Rainie and I managed to laugh it off. But it could have been a lot worse. Once you send a wireless message or photo, it lives forever on social media and search engines, not to mention on another's mobile device. Technology leaves little room for error.

For the all the hours we spend each day emailing, texting, posting, and chatting, we need at least one moment away from the madness. This is a moment to ensure that what you are sending is aligned with what you are feeling, thinking, and living.

## MEDITATE AND CELEBRATE

Embrace the power of 1:11.

Considered a powerful number in numerology and various traditions, 1:11 is a sacred time each day to remember: push back from your desk, take a breath, and reconnect with life.

A reader, Marilynn, wrote me a fascinating email: "[Technology] makes me feel like I should be more connected to people, but really, it's only on a surface level. I gain more from one conversation with a friend than I do from chatting on Facebook for hours. I gain more knowledge from one hike in the woods than I do from reading three hundred articles online."

While the increased connectivity, access to all those articles, and constant communication with others can be a good thing (especially for business), too much technology creates "absence." Absence of time, absence of sensation, absence of peace.

The antidote to absence is presence. It's the feeling you have after a long, sweet nap, or when eating comfort food on a dark, cold night, or when taking a break at 1:11.

Jolie, a schoolteacher, shared with me,

85

"Every afternoon at 1:11 pm, our classroom alarm clock goes off with nature sounds. The children and I stop whatever lesson we're in the middle of, and talk about the beautiful, funny, and delicious things we've noticed during the day.

"I originally started doing it for me, but some of my students noticed the alarm go off at 1:11 and asked what it was for. When I explained your [Happy is the New Healthy] approach, they wanted to participate too. They have taken over the activity!

"Last week, when we returned to school after a field trip, the children noticed what time it was and exclaimed, 'WE MISSED 1:11!' I laughed out loud and told them we could still talk about the moments even though it wasn't the 'right' time.

"It was such a good lesson for me! The pressure of getting everything covered is overwhelming at times, and having the students remind me what's really important is such a blessing."

These are simple solutions to complex problems. When we untangle ourselves from life, we realize posse is just a few letters from pussy, as is love from shove, and breathe from seethe.

At any moment, you are just one deep

breath, one good stretch, and one-glance-at-1:11 away from regaining your clarity and turning an ordinary moment into an extraordinary one.

**Tape this to the side of your computer as a reminder to push back, breathe deeply, and look up:**

*At 1:11, I look to heaven.*

*At 1:11, I look to heaven.*

*At 1:11, I look to heaven.*

# 10
## ~~Lash~~ Laugh Out

**Let That Shit Go!**

I once had a Tai Chi teacher who would say, "As the opponent goes up, he feels you are taller. As the opponent goes down, he feels you are deeper."

If it is a great day and you are catching the breaks, this is the ideal time to be taller. Get out there and make it happen.

If it is a bad day and things are not going your way, go deeper. Let the day pass uneventfully.

But do not force life. That is when you are out of touch with the rhyme and rhythm. That is when you lash out, instead of laugh out.

I produced a few samples of a Yeah Dave Yoga T-shirt to sell at my workshops.

There was a Sanskrit word on the front of the T-shirt that was supposed to mean "to play a musical instrument," because I believe that practicing yoga is like playing the instrument that is your body.

While wearing this Yeah Dave Yoga T-shirt, I was stopped by an Indian man in Union Square in New York City.

"Do you know what that Sanskrit word means?" he said in his Indian accent.

"Yes, it means to play a musical instrument," I told him.

"No, it doesn't. It means to play your musical instrument," he stated firmly.

"So what's the difference? Your instrument, an instrument?" I asked.

The Indian man continued, "You are wearing a shirt that basically translates to mean 'I masturbate.' And if you really want to get specific with your Sanskrit, it actually says, 'When I masturbate, God will come.' "

He continued, "I don't think you intended to say that but you should know it's a terrible thing to have on a T-shirt."

Whoops!

I quickly thought back through the list of approximately ninety people who had purchased one of these shirts, and unknowingly disseminated the message "I masturbate" into the world.

The people who bought these Yeah Dave Yoga T-shirts ranged from schoolteachers and coaches to executives and lawyers, even a rabbi.

God knows where they have worn these shirts . . . and bless the souls of those who actually understand Sanskrit. They must have covered their mouths in disgust upon seeing an upstanding mother of two, member of the country club, head of the PTA, leaving the 10 a.m. power yoga class with her fancy mat bag, Lululemon pants, and a t-shirt saying "I masturbate."

After reaching out and apologizing to as many of these lawyers, doctors, upstanding mothers, and schoolteachers as possible, I looked up on the Internet "damage control after offending people."

That's when I discovered that "being offended" is a section in a popular blog called Stuff White People Like.

As the blog states, "There are few things white people love more than being offended."

Political commentator Bill Maher wrote an Op-Ed for *The New York Times:*

"When did we get it in our heads that we have the right to never hear anything we don't like? . . . I don't want to live in a country where no one ever says anything that offends anyone. That's why we have Canada. That's not us."

Agreed!

I was not going to feel badly about my botched T-shirts. We all make mistakes.

There is a choice we make in life. Either you get offended, or you have a sense of humor. One is a lot healthier than the other. I am not going to say which one. But I will say that the following is something you will never see in the eulogy of an old and contented soul:

"Ronald passed away yesterday at the age of 102. He lived a long, happy life. He ate lots of chocolate, exercised daily, and was easily offended."

## MEDITATE AND CELEBRATE

Think of something or someone who offended you. Now roll with the punch and get over it!

If a roll of toilet paper represented the five-billion-year history of our planet, the existence of humans on the planet would only be .1 millimeter of a square of toilet paper. One human life lasts just a fraction of a second on the cosmic calendar.

We are here for such a short time. Don't waste your life protecting your pride when you can spend that energy enjoying your journey.

Let that shit go!

As author Don Miguel Ruiz said, "Personal importance, or taking things personally, is the maximum expression of selfishness because we make the assumption that everything is about me."

**Remember:**

*What life diminishes, laughter replenishes.*

*What life diminishes, laughter replenishes.*

*What life diminishes, laughter replenishes.*

# 11
## Strike a (Better) Deal with God

### Flex Your Faith Muscle

On the Alaska trip with my brother, in addition to river rafting, we tried an afternoon of halibut fishing with fifteen other tourists. If you grow up fishing, it is part of everyday life. But for two urbanites from L.A., fishing requires a trip with a guide.

So guided we were, on a two-hour boat ride into Resurrection Bay off the coast of Seward, Alaska. It was a crystal clear morning. Sixty degrees, snow-capped mountains, a fantastic cup of morning coffee. And then . . .

It started as a slow drip of uneasiness, with intermittent moments of "I can handle this, no biggie" and then "breathe, breathe, breathe."

When the first waves of nausea started, I tried to use my teachings to keep my brother calm: "The boat is gonna drop anchor, and everything is gonna smooth out and we're gonna be fine. Just breathe."

For the next four hours, my brother leaned off the side of the boat and became a multicolored organic fountain.

I hid in a corner of the boat and got down close to the ground. When I get nauseous, I try to strike deals with God.

"God, seriously, I'll be celibate, I'll eat purslane and drink green juices all day long, I'll become a rabbi, make this nausea go away and I will be your servant day and night, now and forever!"

On and on I went, breathing, ranting, pleading, but the nausea got worse.

We were in dire agony. My brother and I begged the guides to take us back.

But the tour guides refused. "There are thirteen other people on this trip. They paid good money. You just have to wait."

So we waited. For two long hours, bobbing up and down, and up and down, and up and down, and did I mention . . . up and down . . . on a choppy Resurrection Bay.

For those two hours, we felt helpless, weak, sick, and dehumanized. Finally, we started moving on the two-hour trip back to Seward. It was too rough to lean over the edge of the boat, which explains the unforgettable memory of my brother, holding onto a pole, standing upright, shaking his head back and forth. With nowhere to go but out his mouth and down his shirt, the vomit dripped, drooled, and flowed.

It was so awful that all I could think of was the band Widespread Panic singing these lyrics: "All. Time. Low! All. Tiiiime. Loooooow!!"

The second we stepped off that boat and onto dry land, we felt better.

Along with the physical revelation (no more fishing boats), came a spiritual one. In a moment of desperation (which was so minor compared to people who are hungry, sick, and dying), I pleaded with God. Why only in this kind of moment did I think to open up a divine dialogue?

When my own faculties and abilities failed me and I needed to tap into something greater, I was begging, not praying. My faith muscle was flabby.

One of my favorite yoga teachers, Bryan Kest, often teaches how to stretch your feet, which, by the way, is so painful. He explains, "They don't make a machine at the gym to work out your toes. Because it doesn't look good to have strong toes. But let me tell you, if you have unhealthy feet or hurt toes, it's the most painful thing in the world. The resilience of the web depends on the strength of every strand."

So it is with the faith muscle. It will not help you look better, but on the dark days, the sad days, the long days, you need it.

As my Grandma was nearing the end of her life, she struggled like many old people do. Whether falling down in the bathroom or becoming short of breath, she would turn as white as a ghost, afraid that this was it, her final moment.

She never really developed her faith muscle, and in those moments of uncertainty, she was like a basketball player out of position, unsure what to do, where to look, how to be.

Marianne Williamson calls prayer "constant communication with God."

This does not have to mean dropping to your knees at all hours, but what about something as simple as a daily thank you for all that is good in your life?

The ancient teachings say that if you take one step toward God, He will take ten steps toward you.

As I learned in Alaska, it is hard to "step" anywhere with a flabby faith muscle on a rocking fishing boat.

Flex your faith muscle.

If you can tap into your faith in times of comfort, it will be that much easier to access it in times of struggle.

Take a moment today to open your mind, your heart, your body to something greater than your own ego, desires, and thoughts. Some call it prayer. What does prayer mean to you?

Søren Kierkegaard said, "The function of prayer is not to influence God, but rather to change the nature of the one who prays."

Next time you are in a tough spot, whether nauseous on a fishing boat, or God forbid, sick in a hospital, or dare I say, approaching your final breath (as we all will), let us hope for the strength that we may flex our faith muscle with the grace of a warrior, rather than the desperation of two urbanites from L.A. on a rocky fishing boat in Alaska.

**When you need to call upon your faith, consider this prayer:**

*I invite the Intelligence around me*
*to become the intelligence within me.*

*I invite the Intelligence around me*
*to become the intelligence within me.*

*I invite the Intelligence around me
to become the intelligence within me.*

# 12
## Make Peace
## with the Weather

**"In the Fight Between You and the Universe, Back the Universe."**
**Frank Zappa**

One sleepless night, I pulled a Shel Silverstein book off my shelf. I had not read his quirky, catchy, beautiful children's poems in twenty years. It inspired me to write my own Shel Silverstein-esque poem based on someone I know (and love) who always complains about the weather.

Sally Sally hated the snow.
"It always makes my eyebrows glow!"

Sally Sally moped in the rain.
"My feet get wet, then I feel pain!"

Sally Sally seethed in the sun.
"I get so tired, then I can't run!"

Sally Sally cried in the breeze.
"Those allergies, they make me sneeze!"

She cursed at the sky, flicked off the sleet.
She kicked at the clouds, whined in the
    heat.

But day after day, she watched the news.
"Here's the forecast with Jonny Pontews.

"C'mon Jonny, I'm waiting for you.
Say something good, come on through!"

"Hello folks, your forecast tonight
is crystal clear, not a cloud in sight.

"A full moon above, radiant light,
So crazy bright, you could fly a kite!"

"Heck." said Sally, "The moon makes me
    nuts.
That weatherman is a gosh darn putz."

She tried Seattle, "Way too cold!"
Then Delray Beach, sweat through her
    clothes.

To Tucson she leaped, rented a spread,
but desert summers made her feel dread.

She tried some yoga, to lift her frown,
Then told the teacher, "Turn the air down!"

She found a church, dropped to her knees.
The air was too damp. She had to leave.

Finally one day, she had enough,
"Oh God, Oh God, you are so tough!

"First comes the rain, then comes the snow,
what's next, a tornado?"

And at that moment, as you might guess,
down came the thunder, a great tempest.

Sally Sally, she stomped and cried,
"Thunder, oh no! I hate the surprise!"

BOOM BOOM BOOM and a flash so bright,
the lightning came, blinded her sight.

It lit Sally up, head to toe.
What happened, she never did know.

But Sally Sally, she walked away,
whispering, "What a beautiful day."

## MEDITATE AND CELEBRATE
Do you remember that *Saturday Night Live*
skit from the early 80's called The Whiners?

An annoying couple whined about crowded airplanes, whined about waiting at a restaurant, whined about food in the hospital. It is as relevant today as it was over thirty years ago.

We all whine about something. A job. An injury. A relationship. But whining about the weather is the tipping point. That's when the whining goes from a normal human habit to self-defeating behavior.

Make peace with the weather. Is there any other choice?

Next time you are grappling with a freezing winter day or a humid summer night . . .

Harmonize with the heat. Chill in the cold.

Relish the rain. Savor the snow.

Whether it is the weather, the aging process, or something mundane like a broken washing machine, try taking a gentler attitude toward those things over which you have little control.

**Next time you find yourself whining and complaining, gently repeat:**

*Release and Relax.*

*Release and Relax.*

*Release and Relax.*

# 13
## Just Ask a
## 70,000,000-Year-Old

### Carpe the Heck
### Out of Your Diem!

For many years, I have shared Yoga + Chocolate workshops with thousands of people around the world. Only once did I receive a very stern reprimand:

*"Dave:*

*Seriously you need to know what your Yoga + Chocolate workshops do to people. First you relax them, and then you pump sugar into their system which causes insulin resistance, leads to liver disease, and is highly addictive. Yoga and Chocolate should not be considered a wellness event. You've been doing this long enough. Time for change brother Dave."*

I pondered this message and thought back to hiking the Grand Canyon with my wife and her family over the holidays. Let me just say, my in-laws are fitness champions. They run marathons, triathlons, ultra marathons, and megathons. So you can imagine they were motoring up and down the Grand Canyon.

And I, for lack of better words, tend to hike "chocolate-style." I was lagging behind, consumed with the challenge. Despite my exhaustion, I had to keep reminding myself, "Dave, look up. It's only the Grand freakin' Canyon surrounding you in every direction! Hello!"

As it goes when hiking the Grand Canyon, you see things you normally do not see, on the outside and the inside. Lessons become clear that previously were not.

Society and technology have advanced exponentially in the past few hundred years. In the 1800's, people rode steam locomotives instead of hybrid cars, and were excited about basic electricity, let alone watching TV on a mobile device. In the 1700's, people rode horses instead of trains and a candle was the only source of light. I will not pretend to know what life was like in the 1600's. But when someone from the 17th, 18th, or 19th century ventured into the Grand Canyon, they saw the exact same formations, vistas, nooks, and crannies that we see in the present day. Three or four hundred years are a mere flash in the extensive seventy million year timeline of the Grand Canyon.

I finished that hike with a strong note to self. "If you only are here for a flash, you better make it count! Stop worrying so much about how you look, what you eat, and how much money you earn. You are journeying through an exotic place (Earth) with canyons, oceans, and mountains. Experience, taste, indulge! Do NOT deprive."

It is a common message that we hear from yoga teachers, greeting cards, and Oprah specials. But sometimes it really hits you, whether in the majesty of the Grand Canyon or the normalcy of a weekday morning.

On one such morning, I asked a coffee shop owner for the password to their WIFI network. He responded, "The network is called 'why don't you get outside and enjoy this beautiful summer day!"

Here I was getting reprimanded for not living in the moment, and I write books and give speeches about the subject!

After one of these speeches, a man from the audience approached me. "I so badly want to be that guy who is always present. But how?"

Great question. How do you (how do I) become the one with the strength and wherewithal to look up and enjoy the journey? The average person spends almost three hours each day staring at their mobile device. The head-down-thumb-swiping-across-the-screen position is so common that the New York City authorities have strategically placed the words "LOOK UP" on crosswalks to prevent "textwalkers" from getting hit by cars

It is a sign of our times that we are looking down, not just on the streets, but in our stumbling quest for meaning and purpose. Changing this behavior will not come from reading a self-help book or taking a great yoga class. We have to go deeper.

Take a moment to sit with the following questions:

How do you want to be remembered?

Whose life have you impacted deeply?

Have you shared your secrets and gifts with another who can continue your legacy?

Have you dared to dream your greatest dream?

If you could be present at your own funeral, what eulogy would you hope to hear?

There are no prerequisites to living a deeper and richer life. Wherever you happen to be right now, the cozy confines of your bedroom, the airport lounge, or a majestic national park, open your heart . . . and eyes. The treasures are in this moment!

And might I add, to the aforementioned detractor seeking the end of my chocolate-inspired yoga experiences, you will never hear in a eulogy: 'And thank God she stopped eating chocolate!'

## MEDITATE AND CELEBRATE

There's something strikingly similar about being very old, or very young. They both share a certain kind of wonder, a closeness to the Hereafter, whatever that may be.

So next time you are charging too hard through life, and you need that reminder to carpe the heck out of your diem . . .

If you do not have access to the Grand Canyon, here is an alternative:

Ask a five year old, "What's the secret to life?"

My friend's five year old son, who calls me Yahoo Dave instead of Yeah Dave, answered, "More people should play with Legos and trains."

Yes! Yes! Yes!

**Today, dig deeper, live greater, and repeat:**

*This is my time. This is my moment.*
*I celebrate life NOW.*

*This is my time. This is my moment.*
*I celebrate life NOW.*

*This is my time. This is my moment.*
*I celebrate life NOW.*

# 14
## UNLEASH YOUR GENIUS

### STAND ATOP THE TALLEST PLACE IN YOUR MIND

I was taking a class with a teacher at my local gym. She was a lot younger and had a mystique of coolness.

"Loved your workout!" I told her. "Fantastic!"

"Thanks. I was nervous because there was so much people," she responded.

Ooh.

Bad grammar. I let it pass.

"You'll be seeing me again," I told her.

"Thanks, what is you name?" she asked.

She did it again, saying "you name" instead of "your name." Maybe she was from overseas? Or just a hard core New Yorker?

"My name are David," I told her, trying to speak in her "lingo."

Not a good idea. If a conversation could be described by a scent, ours shifted from "sage-inspired-après-yoga-mood-lifter" to "upper-deck-men's-bathroom-at-a-Raiders-game." She may not have been grammatically inclined, but she was sharp. After picking me apart with a look from hell, she gracefully turned and walked away.

So it goes with generation gaps. Certain things fall through the cracks.

*Forbes* magazine reported, "Younger employees are bringing the vernacular of emails, Twitter messages and casual conversations into the office."

And *The Wall Street Journal* mentioned a recent survey taken in 2012, in which 45 of employers percent said they planned to increase training programs to improve employees' grammar and other skills.

Good luck with that.

As I learned in my encounter with the fitness teacher, the type of people who walk around telling you to "mind your p's and q's" are generally the type who hear a lot of "f's" and "you's."

The greatest wordsmith of all, Shakespeare, said, "action is eloquence," something seen so clearly in the above-mentioned yoga teacher's awesome workout.

To each her own expression of life.

If you can't sing, then write. If you can't

write, then paint. If you can't paint, then run. Get it out of you!

And let there be no doubt, you have a spectacular gift, your unique genius to share with the world.

You may not yet have discovered your hidden genius because our world is backward in the way we determine intelligence. According to the ancient Sufi poets, intelligence was based on one's appreciation of music, not career status or IQ. The ancients were onto something.

Psychologist Howard Gardner reports nine types of intelligence:

— Naturalist intelligence (botanist)
— Musical intelligence (violinist)
— Logical-mathematical intelligence (engineer)
— Existential intelligence (yoga teacher)
— Interpersonal intelligence (politician)
— Bodily-kinesthetic intelligence (athlete)
— Linguistic intelligence (writer)
— Spatial intelligence (architect)

You are brilliant in one of the aforementioned ways, and there is a good chance you have been stuffed in the wrong box. As Einstein said, "Everybody is a genius. But if you judge a fish by its ability to climb a tree, it will live its whole life believing it is stupid."

If you are feeling less than smart around your friends or coworkers, speak about what you love. Love is superior to intelligence.

If you feel as if you lack the skills to thrive, explore your passion. Skill is important, but passion is invincible.

If you are insecure about your education or experience, follow the feelings rather than the facts. Joseph Campbell said, "People say that what we're all seeking is a meaning for life. I don't think that's what we're really seeking. I think what we're seeking is . . . the rapture of being alive."

We see rapture in those who have dialed into their particular intelligence, and we see power in those who share it with the world. Like the trainer who gives a great workout and has bad grammar, or the author with beautiful words and bad etiquette, or the mom with strong parenting skills and bad style, each of us has a unique skyline, but only some of us have the audacity to stand atop the tallest place in our mind.

### MEDITATE AND CELEBRATE
Unleash your genius. It's a three step process.

# 1. Declare Your Genius

Get to know your particular genius (aka intelligence) on an intimate level. For instance, the aforementioned fitness teacher is a bodily-kinesthetic genius. She knows it and she lives it! It takes boldness and reflection to know yourself and live that truth every day.

A few years ago, I put a lot of time and effort into designing the business plan for a mobile app. I presented the plan to a friend who listened intently.

Afterward, I expected him to say, "Great presentation, awesome business plan! I love it. I'm investing."

Instead, he said, "This is not right. You are trying to be a CEO. You're not a CEO. You create, you write, you dream. But CEO? No way."

I was mad. How could he say that? I had worked so hard on this presentation.

But he was right. I was not in alignment with my particular genius.

It took some serious soul-searching to get back on track.

Now, I make it a practice to unabashedly declare my genius every day and ensure that I am in alignment.

## 2. Declare Your Weakness

It is equally important to develop an intimate relationship with your weakness, that subject or feeling that makes you tremble. Whether your weakness is related to the body, money, trust, or love . . . move into it, feel it deeply, call it by name.

Consider Daniel Tammet. He is autistic and has a splinter ability to learn new languages in a week, do complex calculations in a matter of seconds, and memorize numbers that are 22,000 digits long. His brain is a wonder of the world. Yet Daniel Tammet has weaknesses. For instance, he struggles to take a simple walk on the beach because he obsesses over the grains of sand, which he feels compelled to count.

Instead of spending his days on the beach, he focuses on his brilliance. He has written several bestselling books and speaks to audiences all over the world.

Daniel Tammet reminds us that weakness is merely a shadow.

Obsession is the shadow of intelligence
Anxiety is the shadow of creativity.
Worry is the shadow of trust.

### 3. Make a Choice

Once you have your bearings and you are deeply familiar with what stands before you (genius) and what stands behind you (weakness), you will be faced with a choice. This is a choice we make moment by moment, hour by hour, day by day. It is a choice to turn from the shadow to the light.

We face this choice every time we feel insecure, every time we replay old patterns, relive old frustrations, rewind to previous losses.

**Next time you are facing this choice, repeat these words:**

*With boldness I climb*
*to the peak of my mind.*

*With boldness I climb*
*to the peak of my mind.*

*With boldness I climb*
*to the peak of my mind.*

# 15
## TAKE VITAMIN P

### POSITIVITY CHANGES EVERYTHING

We hear about "The Universe" from our spiritual teachers, self-help authors, and woo-wooey friends. But rarely do we experience the power of the universe firsthand.

And then a fifty-foot meteor drops into the atmosphere at 30,000 mph and releases 500 kilotons of energy (as in the Ural Mountains of Russia in February 2013), and suddenly we remember the universe. And we realize the universe speaks a different kind of language that includes words like "kiloton" and "megaton."

It requires a certain level of consciousness to harness this massive power. We see it in the Gandhis, the MLKs, the Mother Theresas and those lesser known but equally powerful souls who love so deeply that they penetrate your being. David Hawkins writes in his book *Power vs. Force,* "Only .4 percent of the world's population ever reaches this level of evolution of consciousness." But it is possible. And if you can dial it in, you are playing a different kind of game, and all the rules change.

I was preparing for my morning run, standing at the corner of St. Mark's Place and 2nd Avenue in New York City.

Next to me was a Latino man, on his way to work. "It's cold," I uttered in the bitter morning air.

I don't think he spoke English.

So I said, "Hace frío. Mis pezones son duros," which means "It's cold, my feet hurt." (I majored in Spanish in college and, every so often, I like to test my chops.)

A warm smile melted the Latino man's face. And then he laughed hysterically. With a thick Queens accent, he said, "Bro, you had me at nipples."

It turns out that I did not say in Spanish, "It's cold and my feet hurt," but rather, "It's cold and my nipples are hard." Since eighth grade, I have always confused "pezones" with "pies," the correct Spanish word for feet.

While mildly amusing, this encounter was also a flash of clarity, an intersection of meaning, in which I had a startling revelation.

I had recently spent time with a friend who plays the stock market and watches Detroit sports (not for the faint of heart). In the middle of our conversation, this friend asked, "Have you read the latest Joel Osteen?"

This totally caught me off guard. I would never, ever imagine this friend to be even remotely interested in Joel Osteen, the highly charismatic televangelist who converted a former NBA arena into his personal megachurch.

He told me something he learned while reading Osteen. "You have to ask for what you want. You really have to ask for it, very, very specifically."

So I read deeper into Osteen's simple interpretations of ancient teachings. He shares this story, which I will summarize:

A prophet sees a blind man and says to the blind man, "What do you want me to do for you?"

The blind man says, "I want my eyesight."

So the prophet touches his eyes, and for the first time, the blind man is able to see.

But knowing he was blind, why did the prophet not just heal him? Why did the blind man have to ask?

As Osteen explains, imagine that prophet is standing before you asking the same thing that he asked this blind man. "What do you want me to do for you?"

The way you respond is going to determine what the universe does.

Often we will say, "I just need to pay my electric bill" or "Just help me get over this cold."

Instead, dare to speak in overwhelmingly positive terms: "Please grant me great abundance and financial freedom!" or "Please let vitality and crazy, awesome health flow through my veins."

If you want to communicate with someone including the universe, you have to speak in the language of kilotons and megatons, not "pay my electric bill" or "help me get over this cold."

So today, in your ordinary routine when you are washing the dishes, sorting through emails, or waiting in the carpool line, take a moment to plug in and think really big, really positive, really high-vibration thoughts!

Unless you are profoundly well-versed in the language of the universe, you would be surprised how often:

You ask for health
in the language of wealth,
or hope for a break

119

while desiring a steak,
Or try to create ripples
while talkin' 'bout nipples.

### MEDITATE AND CELEBRATE

Take Vitamin P.

You might be wondering, "What's Vitamin P?"

It's the single greatest health tip I have ever heard.

It has the power to instantly change your attitude, alter the chemistry of your mind, and trigger immense healing in the body.

It turns you from a human into a force of nature. P is for Positivity.

By that, I do not just mean dabble in friendliness, or say your hellos and get on with your day. I mean direct the full force of your being to love, peace, and all that uplifts your heart and soul.

In the book *Positivity,* Barbara Fredrickson proves that if one can have three positive experiences for every negative experience, something amazing happens. You reach a critical mass of positive energy, a tipping point that spills into your professional, parenting, and personal life. But three-to-one takes practice. That's why, according to Fredrickson, only 20 percent of Americans have achieved this ratio.

Try it. Every time you think "Oh man, my hair looks bad today," you have to catch yourself and come right back with three positive thoughts. "But it's beautiful outside, and I can't wait for a delicious cup of coffee when I get to work, and the Dodgers won last night!"

If you are down in the dumps, bring positivity to your day. Change the music, watch more uplifting TV shows, kick up the lighting.

If you are in a dark spot in your career, express gratitude for everything. Write complimentary emails, start up happy conversations, share beautiful ideas.

If you are having a hard time with your health, take a little Vitamin P along with your other medications.

There is just something about positivity that touches the soul. Look at Jim Carrey in the movie *Dumb and Dumber.* Everyone remembers this scene:

Jim Carrey: What are my chances?

Lauren Holly: Not good.

Jim Carrey: You mean not good, like one out of a hundred?

Lauren Holly: I'd say more like one out of a million.

Jim Carrey: So you're telling me there's a chance?!!!

"One out of a million" is like the odds of a meteor hitting the earth. When the seemingly impossible happens, we are talking kilotons and megatons of love, healing, peace, and power. And when you are overwhelmingly, unbelievably, incredibly positive, the impossible happens every single day.

**Here is a little something to keep in your back pocket next time negativity gets the best of you.**

*I am Positive, I am Powerful.*

*I am Positive, I am Powerful.*

*I am Positive, I am Powerful.*

# 16
## UNLOCK THE SECRET
## TO THE UNIVERSE

**"TO THE MIND THAT IS STILL, THE WHOLE UNIVERSE SURRENDERS."**
**Lao-Tzu**

I opened up a major health publication and read the warning signs for anxiety disorders.

— Excessive worry (that's me)
— Sleep problems (oh yeah)
— Irrational fears (all the time)
— Muscle tension (my neck needs a crack NOW)
— Chronic indigestion (not as bad since I went gluten-free, but I did take heartburn medication for ten years)
— Stage fright (does this include social anxiety? If so, then hell yeah!)
— Self-consciousness (OMG yes)
— Panic (only when I can't find my wallet, like every morning)

Maybe you can relate to these symptoms?

Almost 100 million Americans are struggling with anxiety, so you are not alone in feeling like the sky is falling.

Before you fear for your sanity, here is a little Native American vocabulary. The Hopi Indians had a word, Koyaanisqatsi, which means "life out of balance." It is an ancient word to describe an ancient condition. People have had anxiety since the beginning of time. Back then, it was less prevalent.

Now it seems like everyone has anxiety. And this Hopi word implies the key to healing this massive health issue: restore balance and connect with the natural rhythms of life.

Another Native American tribe said it so beautifully, "It's time to stop living on the earth and start living with the earth."

So how do we do this?

A few years ago, I went to a Jack Johnson concert. He came on stage in a t-shirt and jeans with his guitar and a stainless steel water bottle. Here was a huge star performing at an elegant venue, yet he dressed for a campfire on the beach. His casual vibe set the tone for his acoustic folk-inspired music. But there was something about that water bottle, the simplest detail, that said, "I give a shit."

It is the tiniest changes that put you back

in alignment "with the earth." We hear them all the time. But do we embrace them? Why not cancel those thick paper bills that come in the mail when switching to electronic bills is just one click away? Drink your morning coffee in a reusable mug and avoid wasting yet another paper cup. Steer clear of toxic PVC yoga mats and seek out a mat made from earth-friendly materials. If we all adopted one green habit, the world — YOUR world — would be a healthier place.

But even more powerful than going green . . . is going slowly.

In today's world, that's a big favor to ask. We are always moving, always racing, always seeking the next cup of coffee. For God's sake, we even jog in place at a red light to keep our cardio rate up.

In 2009, I started jogging to increase my cardiovascular strength. The little earbud headphones refused to stay in my ears, so I jogged with the giant noise-reducing headphones.

Yes, they were a bit awkward, and I was told that jogging with them gave me a striking resemblance to Warren from the movie *There's Something About Mary.*

One thing I always wondered about: when jogging on streets and coming to a red light, should I stop and let my heart rate decline, or should I jog in place and keep it up?

On a gorgeous, sunny day, I was jogging on a tree-lined street in Santa Monica, California. I stopped at a red light and began to jog in place.

A car of high school kids pulled up at the light next to me. Due to my headphones, I could not hear them, but I noticed out of the corner of my eye that the kids were speaking to me.

Maybe they needed directions? Or maybe they wanted to know if I enjoyed my noise-reducing headphones?

While removing the headphones, I heard one of the high school kids in mid-sentence say, ". . . loser ever!"

"Excuse me, I'm sorry, I couldn't hear you!" I screamed, out of breath while still jogging in place.

"I said you're the biggest loser ever!" the high school kid screamed again.

I wished the light would turn green but it was a slow light. I refused to let these high school kids get the best of me and told them to "Go away!" while continuing to jog in place.

I would have been better off feeding Red Bull to a colicky baby. The high school punks screamed even louder . . .

Then, all of sudden, they got real quiet.

One of the high school kids rolled down the back window and said, "Aren't you my mom's yoga teacher?"

Sure enough, I recognized the kid who had taken my class a few times with his mom.

"Dude, my mom loves your class," the kid said apologetically while shushing his friends in front.

"Does your mom know you're a punk ass bitch?!" I screamed angrily.

The second those words left my mouth, I felt terrible for my slip of tongue.

Jogging in place is awkward, and I was asking for it.


Nowadays, there is no such thing as starting and stopping. We have one speed in life, and that is fast.

We are addicted to this high-intensity life. It's a sociological epidemic.

When waking up, we head straight to our phone or computer and off we go.

When at work, we spend most of the day clicking from email to email and website to website on a connection so fast we no longer complain about it being slow.

When driving, we are navigating the information superhighway on our bluetooth connections and satellite radios.

Faster is better! More efficient is more effective! Convenience rules the modern day!

In some ways, a quicker life is easier.

But there are times when "quicker" suffocates stillness and undermines our connection to the universe. When you are in such a hurry to get to work that you do not have a single minute to enjoy the morning. When you are agitated from too much caffeine and your frantic mind drives you crazy. When you avoid meditation like the plague even though just two minutes of sitting quietly could completely alter the tenor of your day.

Franz Kafka said, "Be quiet, still, and solitary. The world will freely offer itself to you to be unmasked, it has no choice, it will roll in ecstasy at your feet."

If you can take time to unplug and be still, you will awaken to opportunities and synchronicity that are impossible to experience in a frenzied state. That frenzied state forces you to hurry, and make up for whatever you are missing . . . an email, a message, your kid's game, a meeting, a luncheon.

What you are actually missing is the courage to be completely and deeply present, to stop at the red light and forsake pace for peace.

### MEDITATE AND CELEBRATE

Be still.

As goes Lao-Tzu's famous quote, "Nature does not hurry, yet everything is accomplished."

In what way is your life always going and never stopping? Do your days bleed together into one maddening blur? Are your kids growing up way too fast? Are you pounding out emails with barely a moment of rest?

In your pause, savor the opportunity to gather your thoughts, come to your senses, and restore your capacity for enjoying life.

Otherwise, you will just keep jumping from one moment to the next, like one of those ridiculous people whose mind, if not body, is always jogging in place.

**When the pace of life is making you crazy, let these words be your anchor:**

*Stillness is strength.*

*Stillness is strength.*

*Stillness is strength.*

# 17
## GO ALL IN

**HOW YOU DO ANYTHING IS HOW
YOU DO EVERYTHING**

It was the 1985 Encino Little League
Championship Game. I was a less-than-
average player on a very talented team.

Digging into the batter's box in the second
inning, I was nervous, always nervous, and,
on this day, especially nervous.

The stands were packed with a whole cast
of characters: beautiful valley girls with giant hair, awkward teenage kids whose
braces glistened in the hot summer sun, and
those annoying parents who took Little
League way too seriously.

Being a super sensitive kid, I could feel all
the pressure, all the eyeballs, and it was hard
to breathe. During the regular season, I
struck out often and felt the pain each time.
I would go home after a bad game and sulk,
embarrassed and mad for letting my team-
mates down. So in the championship game,

I was white in the face, and sweating out each and every moment.

I stared down the barrel (as they say in baseball) at the tall, lanky pitcher, Eric Rothman. He threw heat (aka fast pitches) and while some kids had real skill, I just hoped for the best when swinging the bat.

I swung hard!

"Strike one!" screamed the ump.

I stepped out of the batter's box, adjusted my protective cup (so uncomfortable), and asked the umpire, "Would that have been a strike?"

"That woulda been way outside, son," he responded.

Yikes, that gave me even less confidence. I had swung at a bad pitch. The pitcher reared back into the windup.

"Strike two!"

It blazed past me.

Two strikes. No confidence. Packed stands. Nervous nelly.

Last chance. I stepped into the batter's box. My heart was pounding. The pitcher looked super confident.

BOOOOOOM!

All I could hear was "Romanelli hits it over the head and GONE! A three-run shot!"

I had hit a line drive home run over the

left field bleachers. I do not remember a single thing about my sprint around the base paths except it was just that: a full-on sprint.

I do remember being back in the dugout in a complete state of shock. I was only twelve. I was thrilled. And I did not think to slow down into a home run trot and celebrate the moment.

A few innings later, I did it again. Another home run, this one to the farthest part of the ballpark in center field. How could it be possible?

After the second home run, once again, I sprinted around the base paths, even faster.

Over the years, I showed the video of these two home runs to friends, roommates, first dates, relatives. More often than not, their reaction included something to the effect of, "That's awesome. But what's with the limp high fives?"

In my sprints around the base paths, I realized, having watched the video eight hundred times, that I doled out a series of very limp high fives. In some cases, I barely touched their hand, and in others I made no contact at all.

Let's get one thing straight. There are no nuances or subtleties about the High Five. You either connect or you do not. Get caught in the middle and you have got yourself a limp high five.

If there is one important lesson I have learned in business, wellness, and life, it is this: do not get caught in the middle. People caught in the middle are mired in mediocrity. They sort of try and sort of don't. They sort of pay attention to their kids and sort of don't. They sort of believe and sort of don't. Such behavior suggests a life half-lived.

If you are going to celebrate, then celebrate! Take the moment by storm. Savor the chocolate! Hug with your body and not your hands. Connect on the high five!

How you do anything is how you do everything.

### MEDITATE AND CELEBRATE
Go all in!

Whether it is how you celebrate, how you pay attention at a meeting, or how you love your kids, if you are going to be there, be there fully.

If you are giving your partner only partial commitment, can you dig deeper?

If you are just going through the motions during your workout, can you give more?

If you are showing up at work with a bad attitude, can you change the energy?

133

It is never a question of if you have what it takes or if you are blessed or if you can do it. The question is if you will claim your blessings, own your power, and rise to the occasion that is your life.

My friends showed me their daughter's high school graduation speech. She stood at the podium and bared her soul to her classmates. She told of how she hid her body in her early days of high school by dressing in baggy sweatshirts and old jeans. And then she started hanging out with the right crowd, who were beautiful "because they thought they were beautiful."

She ended emphatically, "I *decided* I was pretty. I *decided* I deserved to be pretty!"

And that is what it means to rise to the occasion, to show up fully, to go all in.

**When you are stuck in the middle, and mired in mediocrity, repeat:**

*I live, I love, I honor my role with all my heart and all my soul.*

*I live, I love, I honor my role with all my heart and all my soul.*

*I live, I love, I honor my role with all my heart and all my soul.*

# 18
## LOSE THE EGO

### HEED THE LITTLE REMINDERS SO YOU CAN AVOID THE BIG ONES

Whether you are a mom looking for her purpose, an advocate on a mission, or a businessperson seeking greater depth, when you commit to a spiritual journey, you are playing by different ground rules. In the spiritual realm, there is no place for ego. If you boast about your "accomplishments" and boost your ego, the universe will break you down, plain and simple.

And if you don't listen, you will get your warning.

A wise person said that first the universe will throw a pebble, and if you don't listen, then the universe will throw a rock, and if you still don't listen, then it will throw a brick wall.

At some point, you will be humbled.

In 2010, I had a great start to the year. *The*

*New York Times* featured a full-page spread on my brand new Yoga for Foodies concept. I was riding high and not the least bit surprised to receive an email from a crew filming a documentary about a guru named Kumaré. They wanted to film me teaching yoga to Kumaré, who was traveling through the United States and looking to share his philosophies.

I was thrilled about being included in the movie. What this would do for my brand! Plus, it made me think back to my years as a commercial actor. The day I got a commercial acting agent, I drove around L.A. playing the Chevy theme song "Like a Rock" over and over again.

I took acting classes with Howard Fine, a famous acting teacher who loved my rendition of a redneck Luke Skywalker. Soon thereafter, I was in a Mountain Dew commercial followed by a role as an auto mechanic for Montgomery Ward's auto repair shops. So you could say I had the acting bug. But I was not able to evolve past commercials into TV or movie acting. That takes a certain talent, which I did not have.

But wait!

This invitation to be in a documentary triggered dormant dreams of stardom on the silver screen. I had another chance!

I met the film crew at a coffee shop in Phoenix.

The crew set up their equipment. In walked Kumaré with long black hair, flowing robes, and a wooden cane with an "om" symbol on top of it. He barely spoke English, and I proceeded to spend the hour with him, on camera. I taught him how to high five. We shared our philosophies. I led him in a Yoga + Chocolate workshop. I had a good feeling about this!

A year later, I saw an advertisement for the movie, Kumaré. "Here it is!" I said to my wife.

We both watched the preview, excited for my big screen debut.

The preview started with these words: "The true story of a false prophet."

Huh?

The preview shared how Kumaré is the story of a dude named Vikram from Brooklyn who wanted to see the everyday American's desperation for spiritual guidance. So Vikram dressed up like a guru and traveled to Arizona to see if he could act the part and trick people into believing he had spiritual powers.

In other words, Kumaré was the Borat of the spiritual world. In other words, this was all a practical joke, made into a movie. In other words, I had been punk'd!

Of all the people they could have chosen to interview in this film, they chose me . . . sucker extraordinaire!

If you have ever been "punk'd," you have experienced a range of emotions.

At first, I was infuriated. How could they! I have a brand, an image. And then I was embarrassed. How could I not see through this joker's costume. A guru in downtown Phoenix with a wooden cane bearing a giant om on top?

But I quickly grasped the lesson — a pebble tossed by the universe telling me to tone down the ego.

I blogged about my naïveté to my community by writing, "It soon became clear that this 'guru' was an imposter making fun of suckers like me who buy into the whole guru shtick. I had it comin'."

Not an hour after sending it, I received an email from Vikram himself which said,

Namaste, David!
We were just forwarded your blog about Kumaré. We had assumed you had already heard about the Kumaré film. I would love to discuss the film, and the message with you, if you are interested. We appreciate and value our time spent

with you in Phoenix, and hope that we've made a challenging film that you and other people will appreciate.

Best,
Vikram Gandhi (Kumaré)

A few months later, I watched the movie on cable. It was brilliant! And I was only featured in one very brief scene at the end (Thank God). It could have been so much worse.

But I got the message, a soft reminder to mind my manners and remember that a spiritual journey is about meaning, not accomplishment. One too many executives, actors, or self-proclaimed gurus have not heeded the little reminders. And their giant egos have led to a public demise that was painful to watch.

As the saying goes, "A bad day for the ego is a good day for the soul."

**MEDITATE AND CELEBRATE**
Lose the ego!

As John Randolph Price said, "Until you transcend the ego, you do nothing but add to the insanity of the world."

In 1997, I headed to Beverly Hills to take a yoga class with the legendary Bikram Choudhury. The mirror-walled room was packed with over two hundred yogis.

And there he stood. Shiny body. Balled hair. Little Speedo holding tight. And a microphone. Wow, this is the real deal, I thought. Just like how yoga must be in India.

Minutes passed. Bikram had not yet spoken. I waited and waited. What would one of the most famous yoga teacher's first words be? Surely he would say something poetic. I could only imagine spiritual honey flowing from his lips.

A muscular dude shuffled into class late and found his spot in the back of the room. Bikram zeroed in on this muscular dude and said, "You! You in the back! You look good on outside . . ." He paused. Bikram continued, "YOU SHIT ON THE INSIDE!"

Despite his sharp tongue and controversial ways, Bikram still commands the attention of hundreds of thousands, if not millions of yogis all over the world. Thanks to our overbearing egos and unyielding pride, the only way most of us really learn a lesson is when a shiny man in a Speedo screams at us; or when we feel extreme physical pain; or when our heart is broken into a million pieces. But should we be more humble and attentive, there are other, less extreme ways to learn our lessons: Coincidental encounters. Intuitive hunches. Time spent in relaxation and meditation.

Heed these subtle reminders and soft revelations that are only experienced in a humble state.

**And should your ego bust out of its britches, as they all do from time to time, keep this mantra handy:**

*I lose my ego and gain my soul.*

*I lose my ego and gain my soul.*

*I lose my ego and gain my soul.*

# 19
## SAY THE THREE MAGIC WORDS

**ENJOY YOUR JOURNEY**

Much of what we consider to be human ingenuity was actually inspired by thousands of years of natural intelligence. For instance:

Before there was the camera (lens, focus, film), there was the eye (cornea, iris, retina).

Before there were plumbing and hydraulic systems in machines, there were circulatory systems in mammals.

Same goes for the windshield wiper, an idea which came from the eye lid; the solar panel, which was inspired by a leaf's photosynthesis; and Velcro, which was first seen in a plant called the thistle burr.

But the greatest suggestion of a natural intelligence is the fact that a human baby grows in the womb from one cell to trillions of cells without any human intervention. Our scientists and engineers could never create a baby in a lab from scratch.

So here is the million dollar question: are

you willing to believe there is another form of intelligence greater than your own? Call it God, call it nature, call it the universe, call it what you will. Someone or Something figured out the ultimate storage system, DNA. One gram of DNA (aka a single droplet) can store 700 terabytes of data. To store the same kind of data on hard drives, you would need 233 3TB drives weighing a total of 332 pounds.

But the science is not what pushes me past doubt. I believe in a greater intelligence because it is more fun to believe than not to believe.

When I give my whole heart to belief, I find that things start to change, pulsate, and pop. I sense an underlying perfection, a rhyme and rhythm in life's events, an inter-connectedness adding intrigue to every random encounter.

The natural intelligence that created DNA and the thistle burr also has the answers to your questions. But those answers require you to seek, connect, commune.

The rabbi Lawrence Kushner writes, "Everyone carries with them at least one and probably many pieces to someone else's puzzle. Sometimes they know it. Sometimes they don't. And when you present your piece, which may be worthless to you, to another, whether you know it or not, whether they know it or not, you are a messenger from the Most High."

Almost once a day while walking in New York City, I look up to see that I am on a collision course with some random stranger. Usually I am able to avoid the collision, and we walk our separate ways.

But on a warm June morning, getting off the L Train at 14th Street, my attempt to avoid collision failed miserably. I turned left, she turned right, and BAM! We walked right into each other at high speed.

Thankfully, she laughed, I smiled, and we walked on.

Whoever she was, wherever she came from, what are the odds that the two of us would physically collide at some moment in our lives?

Maybe the natural intelligence caused this collision to save her from an oncoming bicycle delivery man (those guys are nuts). Or maybe it was just another chaotic morning in New York City.

I believe these types of random collisions, oddball moments, strange coincidences, are the details, the fine stitching that connects us to the universe.

It takes a certain soulful style to honor

these details, as one with fashion sense would honor the right shoes to match an outfit, or one with culinary sense would honor the right sauce to match the creation.

In that brief, one-second encounter upon colliding in the subway station, what did I have to say to that complete stranger?

"Enjoy your journey!"

A taxi driver in rural Alaska had recently shared that expression with me. He came up with it after spending six months with his dying father in a hospice. He recalled, "How is it possible that I lived fifty years but did not get close to my dad until his last six months? Do not make the mistake I made. Do not squeeze what should be a lifelong journey into the last six months of life. Enjoy it now."

The woman in the subway station looked back at me. She thought about it, as people often do when hearing those three words.

"Enjoy your journey!"

Try saying it next time you bump into someone. The strange person with whom you just collided might think you are an absolute nut job. But you just may be the missing piece to that person's puzzle. You just might awaken them to the mystery, brilliance, and blessing of simply being alive.

Say the three magic words.

They are a wakeup call, a reminder, that not only are we surrounded by a brilliant universe, but also an abundant one.

Think how many stars are in the sky (100 billion galaxies with 100 billion stars in each), how many cells are in your body (75 trillion), how many times your dog will kiss your face (1,000,000 times) if you let him.

**Next time you see a pharmacist in a lousy mood, a coworker grinding through a stressful day, or a total stranger in passing . . .**

*Enjoy your journey.*

*Enjoy your journey.*

*Enjoy your journey.*

# 20
# WIN A SMALL VICTORY
# FOR YOUR SOUL

## STAND UP FOR THE
## PRESENT MOMENT

The Grateful Dead have Deadheads, the Green Bay Packers have Cheeseheads, Star Trek has Trekkies. And how can we forget . . . Momenteers! That is what I call fans and supporters of the present moment.

We need more Momenteers, more people who advocate showing up and sticking up for the moments that matter most.

It's just like sticking up for your kid getting yelled at by another parent in Little League, or supporting your coworker getting unfairly harangued at a meeting, or most importantly, defending your wife's cooking when it is not duly appreciated.

For anyone who puts in long hours in the kitchen, you know there is no greater reward than appreciation for your hard work, and no greater insult than disrespect for your offering.

Or so I learned when I invited my hippie friend Mike over for dinner.

"Natural" is how I described him to my wife. Mike's distinguishing feature was a fluffy beard which ran the length of his neck.

Some beards are clean, conditioned, combed, but Mike's had its own ecosystem. If you dared to reach your hand into his beard, surely you would find something living, not to mention scraps and shards from Mike's latest jaunt across America following the band Phish. But hey, who's judging?

We sat down for dinner, and I was excited to watch Mike's reaction. When you taste my wife's cooking, it is impossible to be anything but ecstatic! First up was a dish of perfectly layered eggplant, zucchini, and tomatoes from the farmer's market all topped with a buttered herb breadcrumb topping.

"This looks amazing, honey!" I told her.

I placed a plate down in front of Mike, "Bon appétit."

"Thanks. Hey, do you have any ketchup?" Mike asked.

For those of you who painstakingly prepare delicious food, you know that someone asking to pour ketchup on your creation is like asking a friend, "Hey would you rub on my tushie?" It hurts.

"Mike, we don't have any ketchup. Just try it, you'll love it," I told him firmly.

"What about some ranch dressing?" he asked.

Ranch dressing?

That's even worse, as if the friend who asked you to rub on their tushie has breath that smells like a rotting gefilte fish substitute served in an Aeroflot (Russian airline) snack pack.

"Mike, we don't have ranch dressing; trust me, you gotta just try it. Honey, this is sooo good, thank you," I said to my wife, trying to save the day.

"Maybe some mayonnaise? Just a little somethin'?" Mike asked again.

Asking a chef for mayonnaise? That's like gnawing on a chicken wing while stomping on a butterfly in front of a hippie vegan.

Mayonnaise is nuclear.

Mike ended up trying the layered eggplant, zucchini and tomatoes without any ketchup, ranch dressing, or mayonnaise. And he truly enjoyed it.

But nuclear is nuclear. There is absolutely no recovery from a request for mayonnaise. Never was and never will be.

From smartwatches to computerized ski goggles, we are becoming one with our machines. With each day, technology becomes more integrated into our lives. Even the hippiest of hippies like Mike with the fluffy beard uses technology to check Phish's latest set list, redeem the code on their ticket stub to download the concert for free from Phish's mobile app, and watch the live webcast of the Phish concert. Technology is not all bad, but it is definitely not all good.

A cover story of *Newsweek* read "Is the Internet Making Us Crazy?" In this article, Susan Greenfield of Oxford University writes that "digital addiction is an issue as important and unprecedented as climate change." She explains that if we are not careful, we will become a nation of "glassy-eyed zombies."

Before you pick up a pair of computerized ski goggles that project the Internet directly onto your eyeball, please take a moment to consider:

- There are people who can taste the true flavor of life, and there are people who pour ketchup and mayonnaise on fine food.
- There will be the glassy-eyed zombies who depend on the internet on their eyeball for navigation, calculation, and identifica-

tion, and there will be people who look to their intuition, sensory perception, and memory.

Humanity stands at a massively significant fork in our evolutionary road.

It is decision time.

The tidal current of information is about to push you over the edge toward "the singularity," an era where humans and machines are one and the same. We see this movement taking shape all around us. The gadgets are getting smaller; we are wearing technology on our ears, our wrists, soon over our eyes, and eventually in our bodies.

Are we just supposed to be OK with that?

You still have time to crawl out of the rushing torrent of information and Say NO to the mayonnaise, the invasive forms of technology, all that sullies the raw and natural experience, and YES to the true flavor, the sensory-based memories, and all that enhances your humanity!

## MEDITATE AND CELEBRATE

Win a small victory for your soul.

Catch yourself pulling your phone out of your pocket when your attention might be better served enjoying the sunny day.

Be completely present with your kids, even

when you are slammed at work and struggling to concentrate.

Cuddle up with your family instead of retreating to your private corner to play a game on your phone.

These are the small victories that restore the true flavor to the human experience.

Imagine if you woke up one morning and someone said, "Today is going to be a normal day. Everything will be fine. And you will never remember this day ever again."

How uninspiring! And yet, most days are like that. We are slammed from the second we wake up until the very second we fall asleep, without a single memory of the day gone by.

What if that same person said to you, "Today is going to be a normal day. Everything will be fine, except you are going to have one moment that is so incredible, you will never forget it for the rest of your life."

Would you not dive into that day with impassioned curiosity to discover this "unforgettable moment?"

All it takes is one moment, one victory, one bite of layered eggplant, zucchini, and tomatoes (without mayonnaise) to shift the energy from fearing to loving, from dread-ing to dreaming, from grinding to living!

**Keep it simple. I call it the BFD mantra:**

*A beautiful, funny, and delicious (BFD) moment each day keeps the stress away!*

*A beautiful, funny, and delicious moment each day keeps the stress away!*

*A beautiful, funny, and delicious moment each day keeps the stress away!*

# 21
# MAKE IT A BAD HAIR DAY

## IF LIFE IS PASSING YOU BY . . .
## LET IT GO

"Do you want to see it from behind?" the haircutter asked, holding the mirror up so I could see the back of my head.

"I don't even like it in front," I told her.

"What do you mean? It looks great all around."

"C'mon. I look like a gnome," I responded.

It was a bad haircut. It happens to the best of us. But it is never fun to be on the receiving end of your haircutter's hangover.

She stood over me, scissors in hand, trying to figure out her next move.

I just looked at myself, wondering if I could somehow alter my wardrobe to suit this new look. Possibly, if I could incorporate some mesh, eye shadow, and Virginia Slims cigarettes, I could make it work.

"What's a gnome?" the haircutter asked.

"Have you ever seen those SkyMall magazines on the airlines? They sell these small humanoid statues you can put in your garden for decoration. Those are gnomes," I muttered under my breath.

Later that evening when my wife got home, she looked as if I had presented her with a hairless cat (it's called a Donskoy) or a nibbling gerbil.

"No fucking way," was all she said.

"The haircutter screwed up," I told her.

"Who do you think you are, Prince Valiant?"

"Prince Valiant looks better than a gnome," I told her.

"What's a gnome?" she asked, reaching for her phone to get me an appointment with a new haircutter.

This was not the first time I had a bad haircut.

In fact, I had a bad hair era (1985–88). I spent those years chasing cool, pursuing popularity, trying to fit in. As a seventh or eighth grader, I could not find a date in a female prison with a fist full of pardons. But why?

I spent so much time and energy trying to arrange my hair (I used a blow dryer . . .

hello!), wear the right the clothes (I wore white Guess jeans . . . what?), and cover my zits (some were so big they warranted names).

I was always yearning to be somebody I was not.

Here is the question to ask yourself: "If you could choose anyone, would you want to date you?"

When you really love someone (especially yourself), you see past their zits, clothes, and hair. You love their passion, humor, and energy.

If I could go back in time and have a conversation with the seventh and eighth grade version of me, I would say: "Have a bad hair day! Let loose. Be YOU!"

That bad haircut came at just the right time, as if the universe was giving me a little reminder: "relaxing and letting things go is much healthier than tensing up and fitting in."

As I write this, there has been a clique of people with huge followings joining forces and putting together big wellness events.

I admired what they were doing and emailed to ask about being included. I got zero response.

I felt intuitive alarm bells ringing in my

ears: "Been there, done that. Wake up!"

Can you relate? Is there something exclusive going on in your world?

Are you trying to keep up with those crazy fitness people when your body just will not do those things? Are you feeling left out by a certain group of "friends" who did not invite you to the weekend getaway? Is there someone you want to date who will not give you the time of day?

Lesson learned: a bad day (or bad haircut) need not be a bad era.

If it feels like life is passing you by, let it go!

Why walk in someone's else's footsteps when you can walk down your own awesome path.

The Grateful Dead sing it perfectly in the song "Ripple":

There is a road, no simple highway
Between the dawn and the dark of night
And if you go, no one may follow
That path is for your steps alone.

### MEDITATE AND CELEBRATE

Make it a bad hair day.

In any way your hair or job or body type makes you feel frozen out, excluded, or forgotten, turn the other way and start your own trend, have your own party, do your own thing!

Entrepreneur Derek Sivers narrated a video on YouTube showing how to start a trend and be a leader rather than a follower. In this video, there is a shirtless dude dancing alone on a grass field at a live concert. His dance moves are ridiculous, flamboyant, and he cares NOT what anyone thinks. As Sivers says, "The lone nut braves ridicule."

Another guy starts dancing next to "the lone nut." Sivers calls this guy the first follower. Then a second follower joins and "three is a crowd and a crowd is news." In a matter of seconds, they reach a tipping point. Three people become twenty people and then one hundred people and the lone nut suddenly has started his own mini-movement of crazy dancers.

A lone nut teaches us the same lesson over and over again.

If you are not your own rabid, loyal, diehard fan, why would anyone else be?

**Whenever you are feeling left out or left behind, repeat this saying:**

*Awesome. Feeling it, living it, dreaming it.*

*Awesome. Feeling it, living it, dreaming it.*

*Awesome. Feeling it, living it, dreaming it.*

# 22
## OWN YOUR SUPERPOWER

**LOVE IS AN UNSTOPPABLE FORCE**

The following is a famous conversation between Gandhi and Paramahansa Yogananda, widely credited with being the first person to introduce yoga to the United States in the 1800's.

Yogananda: Please tell me your definition of [the Sanskrit word] "ahimsa."

Gandhi: The avoidance of harm to any living creature in thought or deed.

Yogananda: Beautiful ideal. But the world will always ask, may one not kill a cobra to protect a child, or one's self?

Gandhi: I could not kill a cobra without violating two of my vows–fearlessness, and non-killing. I would rather try inwardly to calm the snake by vibrations of love. I cannot lower my standards to suit my circumstances.

This was coming from a man who had an appendectomy without anesthesia to prove that he could separate his mind from his senses.

This was coming from a man who slept next to nubile, naked women to test his restraint.

This was coming from a ninety pound man who single-handedly overcame the British Empire, which was then the greatest force in the world.

Let's take the man for his word and assume, if Gandhi had come face to face with a cobra, he would have used the power of love to overwhelm it.

The greatest humans to have walked the earth have known that love is the highest frequency, the strongest response, the ultimate form of offense and defense.

Many of us use love on offense. We seek love, we celebrate love, we express love.

But what does it mean to use love as defense?

I boarded the plane bound from Chicago to Los Angeles. We taxied down the jetway, waiting for takeoff. The pilot announced that the air conditioning unit was malfunctioning, and we needed to return to the gate. To make matters worse, everyone was asked to disembark so the plane could be repaired. Ugh!

As we unhappily waited in the terminal for over an hour to reboard, a sweaty man with a toupee lost his patience and went bananas on the poor United Airlines customer service agent.

Most everyone in the vicinity remained paralyzed, watching, unsure what to do. The poor customer service agent, exhausted and overworked, sat there and took the abuse.

But then, in a beautifully courageous act that deserves some kind of citizen's medal of honor, one man jumped in on behalf of the poor customer service agent. And then another man jumped to her defense. And before you knew it, four people were backing down the sweaty man with a toupee.

That is love on defense!

That is how Gandhi took down the British Empire. And that is how these four strangers helped an innocent woman at Chicago O'Hare.

Love is the one real superpower. And I do not use that word lightly.

On April 11, 1982, in Lawrenceville, Georgia, Tony Cavallo was in the driveway fixing his car. Suddenly the jack collapsed, and Tony was knocked unconscious and pinned under the car. His mother, Angela Cavallo, came to the rescue and lifted all three thousand pounds of the car off her son, while a neighbor pulled him to safety.

Another example occurred on March 2, 2012. Stephanie Decker used her body to shield her two children from the 175 mph winds of a tornado in Henryville, Indiana. Stephanie suffered a punctured lung, seven broken ribs, and two crushed legs — both of which later had to be amputated. Remarkably, her two kids did not suffer a single scratch.

If you are wondering if you have what it takes to help another, to overcome an obstacle, to be stronger than your problems and greater than your circumstances . . . call upon love.

*A Course in Miracles* states, "And what you call with love will come to you. Love always answers."

## MEDITATE AND CELEBRATE
Own Your Superpower.

Whatever the scenario, love has the power to overcome.

Dr. Dean Ornish, founder of the Preventive Medicine Research Institute, said, "I am not aware of any other factor in medicine that has a greater impact on our survival than the healing power of love and intimacy. Not diet, not smoking, not exercise, not stress, not genetics, not drugs, not surgery."

Love may be all-powerful, but it does not always come easily. When we are really sick, mad, jealous, or stressed, it takes a lot of strength to make a loving choice. We need a method, a means by which to draw from the heart when we would just as soon cuss our fate.

The legendary superheroes have a go-to move by which they unleash their superpower. Superman rips open his shirt to reveal the "S" before he flies off and saves the day. And Diana Prince spins around in circles to shed her civilian attire and become Wonder Woman. There is great symbolism in their moment of transformation.

Mantra offers that same transformation, shifting your attention backward toward the power of love.

**Next time you feel anger, jealousy, stress, or sickness . . . call upon the ultimate superpower by repeating these words:**

*Love above me.*
*Love below me.*
*Love around me*
*Love within me.*

*Love above me.*
*Love below me.*
*Love around me*
*Love within me.*

*Love above me.*
*Love below me.*
*Love around me*
*Love within me.*

# 23
# HELP AN OVERWHELMED MOM

**"THERE ARE NO FIXTURES IN NATURE. THE UNIVERSE IS FLUID AND VOLATILE."**
**Ralph Waldo Emerson**

John Evans was the oldest man in the world when he passed in 1990 at 112. He attributed his longevity to a regular pattern of sleeping and eating, including a morning drink of hot water with a touch of honey.

Shigechiyo Izumi, purportedly 120 years old when he died, drank barley wine every single day.

Routines can be good. They provide a comforting consistency. But routines are better when mixed with a little sugar and spice. Jeanne Calment lived to be 122 and ate two pounds of chocolate each week. Calment said laughter was her secret to longevity, "I could never wear mascara, I cried too often when I laughed."

There is a fine line between routines that

provide a healthy foundation, and those with the ill effect of numbing our capacity for life. Whether driving to work on the same road year after year or eating the same breakfast every single day, such routines can erode our sanity.

Ask yourself:

Are you willing to leave the office and miss a few emails on your lunch break for the chance to bask in the summer sun?

On the evening walk with the dog, would you dare to take a different route and see what's shakin' a few streets over?

As author Alice Walker wrote, "I think it pisses God off if you walk by the color purple in a field somewhere and don't notice it."

On that note, would you change up your morning commute in order to drive by those stunning purple flowers in full bloom?

We all have routines. When I travel, I must keep things very regimented: I get to the airport two hours early; wash my hands right away; wait in the security line; find a cup of hot coffee; look at *Sports Illustrated* and *National Geographic* in the store; wash my hands again; and head to the gate. When the airline attendant begins the boarding process, I double check that I have my ticket and mindlessly walk down the jetway while checking emails on my mobile device.

On one such mindless jaunt down the jetway, while trying to bang out an email on my phone, I heard a woman complain, "Aren't you gonna say sorry?!"

I looked up and noticed the woman was speaking to me. She was an overwhelmed mom trying to take her baby out of the stroller when I accidentally bumped into her leg.

"I'm so sorry. I totally apologize!" I said.

But the torrent of passengers pushed me down the jetway, and onto the plane.

I thought, "I will never see that lady with the stroller again. That was my one chance to show her who the real Dave Romanelli is. And I blew it! To her, I was not Yeah Dave. I was the jerk in the blue headphones, human being #1,298 who passed by her at JFK."

Such was the effect that all this routine had on my ability to recognize others. How many moments and people have I failed to notice because I was mired in my routines?

When you take time to recognize an overwhelmed mom on the jetway (or don't), that matters.

When you are the one to move your mat in the crowded yoga class and make room for the person who cannot find a spot (or

168

don't), that matters.

When you stop and chat with the barista in your coffee shop (or don't), or talk to the receptionist you always pass by (or don't), or make time to help someone put their luggage into the overhead bin (or don't), that matters.

But it is not just strangers. We become numb (sometimes sadly so) to the ones we love most.

"There goes my husband, in a bad mood, again."

"There's my spouse, lying next to me in bed, frustrated as ever. Same ol, same ol."

"There's my boss, stressed to the bones. Shocker."

What can you do? You can do everything! Take the world by the shoulders. Look the world in the eyes. Tell people who you are and why you care. Otherwise, what's the point? To wake up, have coffee, eat a bagel, go to work, talk about the crazy weather, do a social media post, go home, watch TV, have a moment or two with your spouse and kids, and do it all over again the next day . . . for 30 years?!

There is more to life than that.

When we are defined by our routines, we deny the universe opportunities to reach us. But, when we break free from our routines, we are ripe for revelation.

That slight spark caused by my slight kick sent me on a long 500 mph spiral across America. I spent the whole flight thinking about that lady on the jetway, and lo and behold, on the way off the plane, there she was again, dealing with luggage and her stroller.

I had a second chance.

I said to her, "I want to let you know I'm sorry. I spent the whole flight thinking about how I kicked you and walked right by and that's what's wrong with the world."

I stopped to help her with her luggage while she put her baby into the stroller.

The real tests of character are these rare and fleeting moments when you have the opportunity to bust through the sameness of your routines and share your light with a total stranger.

God knows how many of those tests I have failed in the past.

But on this morning, at least this once, I passed. That matters!

## MEDITATE AND CELEBRATE

Even if it means busting up your routine, help an overwhelmed mom, a pregnant woman who needs a seat on the subway, or an old lady trying to drag her luggage off the baggage carousel.

When you help someone on the jetway, you feel the love in your heart.

When you stand up for someone on the subway, you stand up for yourself, for your own dignity.

When you help an old lady get her luggage, you relieve another's burden, and release your own.

The book *A Course in Miracles* says, "What you give to others you give to yourself."

But this is not just about helping strangers.

The routines of home life can lull you into a malaise that is hard to shake loose. When we know someone well, we might just question whether trying something new is even worth the effort. And that is like asking whether another sunset is really worth watching; or another kiss from your puppy is really worth your time.

When you miss the mom in the jetway, ignore the attention-deprived partner, and forget to enjoy the purple flowers, you take a step closer to death.

When you help the mom in the jetway, love the attention-deprived partner, and pause for the purple flowers, you take a step closer to life.

We make this choice almost every moment

of every day.

**Should you need a wake-up call, repeat these words;**

*I choose change.*
*I choose hope.*
*I choose life.*

*I choose change.*
*I choose hope.*
*I choose life.*

*I choose change.*
*I choose hope.*
*I choose life.*

# 24
# LET LOVE RULE!

**FALL IN LOVE AND SPREAD IT**

To anyone who has lost a loved one, or had a heart broken, or bled angst in the dark days of a long distance relationship, you know the curse of love. It has teeth, and it bites hard. It leaves scars and causes pain.

But if we keep our hearts open, love will return with the magic and power to heal and heal fast. Along with its sharp teeth, love has playful paws, a silky coat, and a mouth that showers us with kisses.

Allow me to introduce you to the happiest dogs I have ever seen. They do not have rich owners.

They are not freshly groomed.

They are not chewing on a juicy bone.

These dogs live and roam with packs of young homeless people who wander the streets of New York City's Alphabet City. As you might imagine, the homeless people are rough around the edges, dirty, broke, and sometimes broken.

But their dogs always surprise me, because they appear to be playful, loyal, and downright happy. They are mixed breeds, usually some pit bull, but rarely vicious, and profoundly obedient to their masters.

I cannot tell you how many times I have walked by a struggling homeless person with their dog nuzzled up against them. It's why humorist Josh Billings wrote, "A dog is the only thing on earth that loves you more than he loves himself."

Sometimes we forget that, in its primal form, a dog's priority is not to be clean and lying on a doggy bed, but to be outside, free, roaming with its pack.

Trying to imprint human behavior on a dog is like forcing our desires on love.

We say or think: *I love her so much; I don't understand why she doesn't love me! He said he's over it, but I will make him love me again!*

These are examples of how we try to wrap our thoughts around love. Mythologist Joseph Campbell once said that the word "amor" (Latin for love) spelled backwards is "roma." He explained that in the Middle Ages, the Roman Catholic church thought it had dominion over love, justifying marriages that were political and social in their character.

Would you want someone telling you who to love and who to marry? That's like coiffing a dog, dressing it in human clothes, and feeding it escargot and rosé wine.

A dog in its most pure form is dirty, hungry, loving, and loyal. And love is the same way, raw in its essence, fiercely resistant, subjecting you to extreme emotions, but also injecting you with a supernatural life force that makes this journey HOT.

So if you spend too much time coiffing the dog called love, consider this.

Set it free! Let it run.

Stop trying to control where it wants to take you, what it wants to show you, who it wants you to know, where it wants you to go. No leashes, no commands, no training, no doggy treats. Trust love, even the part that bites.

Kahlil Gibran said, "For even as love crowns you so shall he crucify you."

Here is the million dollar question: Can you handle that?

### MEDITATE AND CELEBRATE

Let love rule. Trust it completely.

As much as we like to think we have control over love, we do not. For anyone who has fallen in love with a dangerous maiden or a dark dude, you know that love can be incredibly inconvenient, impossibly painful, totally overbearing. And there is nothing you can do about it. You can't turn love on or off.

All we can do is trust love, and open our hearts completely. Author Washington Irving wrote, "Love is never lost. If not reciprocated, it will flow back and soften and purify the heart."

If you are struggling with a difficult marriage, if you are wailing in the pain chamber from a broken heart, if you are feeling rejected and lonely, could it be that you are softening, purifying, detoxing your heart?

Sometimes we need those difficult relationships to clear out the pipes, to help us move through unresolved issues, and to make room in our hearts for the healthy relationships waiting just around the corner.

The sooner you trust love, the sooner love will guide you toward the next chapter, whether that's a new era in a long marriage or a brand new relationship.

**In the midst of love's intensity, remember:**

*When push comes to shove, I trust in love.*

*When push comes to shove, I trust in love.*

*When push comes to shove, I trust in love.*

# 25
## SCHMOOZE LIKE BILL CLINTON

---

**GO STRAIGHT FOR THE HEART**

For good health, try this:

Take a deep breath, relax, and lift the corners of your mouth up. The miraculous smile.

Recently, while making my way through airport security, I heard a TSA employee say, "How come nobody smiles anymore?"

He was onto something. Research shows that babies smile over two-hundred times each day; the average woman smiles sixty-two times each day, and the average man smiles only eight times each day.

We go to great lengths to look beautiful, dress nicely, and renovate our homes and bodies, but if you can't smile, what's the point?

A dour person with a great physique? Booooring.

A frowner with a fancy handbag and designer jeans? Booooooooo.

A long face in a fancy home? Something ain't right!

When I wake up each morning, I have a personal challenge: to smile or say hello to ten people before 10 a.m. In my gritty New York City neighborhood, people are not always in the mood for such overtures. Some folks will look at me as if I shot them in the eye with breast milk from my man boob, when all I said was "Hi" or "Good morning." But some folks smile back, and in those brief two seconds, I understand why comedian Victor Borge said, "A smile is the shortest distance between two people."

It is even more effective when you actually try to converse with someone. Or better yet, how about really getting personal and reading the name off their name tag? Not to say this always works. I tried it once at a local health food market.

"Thank you, Gaetan, I appreciate your help," I said and smiled warmly at the employee working at the local food market.

I pronounced it "Gay-tan."

He looked at me stone-faced and said, "It's pronounced Gay-toe. It's a French name."

So I tried again, "Gay-toe, thank you. I appreciate your assistance."

He corrected me again, "The accent is on the 'toe.' "

I am very non-confrontational, so I said, "Gah-toe, seriously, I'm sorry."

He replied, "It's not Gah-toe, it's not Gay-tan, it's Gay-toe with an accent on the toe. How would you like it if someone called you Gay Dave instead of Yay Dave?"

I was stunned. "First of all, Gay-toe, it's Yeah Dave, not Yay Dave, and how the heck do you know my name?"

"Because Gay Dave, I read your blog. And it SUCKS!"

Clearly, the warmth of a smile, or the attempt to call someone by name, is not always enough.

## THE SECRET SAUCE

Bill Clinton is widely considered one of the most effective communicators in the world. Anyone — and I mean anyone — who has met Bill Clinton will tell you about his otherworldly magnetism and powerful presence. This is a man who smiles and says hello and does so with absolute mastery.

White House intern Sean Stephenson shared some of Clinton's tricks for masterful communication during his years in the White House:

## 1. Clinton Made Physical Contact.

On many occasions, Clinton would place his hand on a visitor's shoulder, back, or forearm to get the person's attention. As mentioned previously, touch is rare. Entire days go by without any physical contact. Just the slightest contact can create instant connection.

## 2. Clinton Told a Story.

Story lifts us out of the swamp by connecting the fragments and igniting the embers of childhood fantasy. We are all suckers for a good story, and we are all desperate to get out of our heads, even for a matter of seconds.

In Hollywood mogul Peter Guber's book *Tell to Win,* he shares Clinton's ability to use story. It was the 1992 presidential campaign. Bill Clinton needed to raise $90,000 at the very last minute to keep his teetering campaign alive. He called Peter Guber, in hopes that he could rally the Hollywood community.

With a donation limit of $1,000 per person, Guber would have to put his own reputation on the line to rally 90 last-minute supporters. He hesitantly asked, "Do you really think you can win?"

Instead of listing off reasons and policies,

Clinton used story to evoke emotion. He asked Guber, "Have you ever seen the movie *High Noon*?"

*High Noon* is the story of an old fashioned Western showdown. The star of the movie, a sheriff named Will Kane, expects the whole community to back him up as he prepares to face off against a bad gang. But only one young boy shows up for the fight.

Nonetheless, Will Kane scraps his way to victory against all odds. It is a Hollywood classic.

In his moment of truth when his campaign was on the brink of collapse, Bill Clinton said to Peter Guber, "This is High Noon."

Being in Hollywood, of course, Guber knew and loved the movie. He was fired up and instantly rallied supporters to keep Clinton's campaign alive.

Clinton became president, and the rest is history.

As Guber recalls, "I don't know if Clinton was actually a movie buff, but he sure knew where to look for story material that would resonate with the Hollywood community."

### 3. Clinton Chose His Words Wisely.

The intern reported that he never caught President Clinton "taking the verbal low road, slinging slang with disregard." He chose his words wisely to communicate just the right message.

It all comes down to making the authentic effort to connect with other human beings. When you cannot read the name on the name tag (hey, you try pronouncing Gaetan), reach out and touch the person on the shoulder, back, or forearm. Tell a story. Smile.

Sometimes we forget that every human life is a vast constellation of memories, friendships, dreams, and defeats. And it takes a certain kind of courage, a certain type of combustion to bust loose from the familiarity of your own existence and enter the mysterious atmosphere of another human being.

That being said, you may burn up on entry, as was the case with Gaetan or those shell-shocked folks in my neighborhood to whom I say hello.

But the alternative to human contact is increasing isolation of the mind. A mind, forced to face flashing screens instead of blinking eyes, may be headed toward a slow and painful demise. And that is so unnecessary when the solution is as simple as flashing your pearly whites.

I once asked a European, "What do you do?"

He told me it was a very rude and very American question. He went on to explain that Americans put so much emphasis on one's profession, when it should be on their passion, beliefs, and style.

It makes perfect sense. Who wants to be identified by a job they may not enjoy?

As a rule of thumb, I will never ask someone what they do during an initial introduction. Instead, I ask what they believe in, what they stand for, who is their favorite musician, if they like ice cream, what is the best burger they ever had . . . anything but "What do you do?"

"What do you do" or "What do you believe in?"

A fake smile or a real smile.

A shallow connection or an honest intention.

The slightest shifts can have the most dramatic impacts

**When you are feeling the need for deeper connections in your life:**

*Go eye to eye, and heart to heart.*

*Go eye to eye, and heart to heart.*

*Go eye to eye, and heart to heart.*

# 26
## MAKE LIKE
## THE MAGIC MONKS

**WITH A BREATH OF LENGTH COMES INVINCIBLE STRENGTH**

Do you remember what you did a week ago Thursday? What about two weeks ago Friday?

Life is a big blur. Who can remember a week ago with any sort of clarity?

But there are rare examples of people who do remember.

On a beautiful July evening in 2013, I met such a person, Ian, who answered the question, "Yes, I do remember last Thursday and two weeks ago Friday."

"OK, fine," I told him. "How about three weeks ago Wednesday?"

"Yes, I was with my girlfriend at an Indian restaurant on 1st Avenue."

He went on to explain that he has synesthesia, a condition that causes a mingling of the senses due to cross-wiring in the brain. In Ian's case, this helps him remember every day of the past six months. How? Ian associated the days with shapes and colors and therefore had an easier time shuffling through his memories.

Other synesthetes (as they are called) associate numbers with shapes or sounds. Approximately 1% of the population has synesthesia, so it is relative rare to meet someone with the condition. And even rarer to meet someone like James Wannerton, who crosses taste and sound.

Wannerton explains that synesthesia affects his romantic attraction. For instance, according to Wannerton, the name Janette sounds like bacon. And Chrissie is strong and salty. He says it would be the equivalent of smell for a normal person (i.e., you would not be able to date someone if he or she smelled badly, just as Wannerton cannot date someone if her name elicits a bad taste).

Does this synesthesia stuff seem a bit farfetched? Scientists believe we may all be "synesthetes" to a certain degree.

Oxford University psychologist Charles Spence has found that normal people tend to associate sweet tastes with high-pitched notes (like the sounds of a piano) and bitter flavors with low notes (like the sounds of brass instruments).

This crossing of sound and taste is a subtle ability we may one day learn to exercise in order to enhance sensory experience. For instance, Spence conducted an experiment in which he had people eat toffee while listening to both high and low notes. He reported, "We were significantly able to change the rating of the bitterness and sweetness of the food depending on the sound they were listening to." In the future, a chocolate shop might enhance the taste of the chocolate by playing certain high-pitched notes over the sound system.

Synesthesia is one of many hidden or rarely accessed abilities of the human brain. Lest we forget, that brain in your head is considered the most complex object ever discovered in the universe. And when watching The Magic Monks, we have to wonder just how many of these hidden abilities are waiting to be discovered?

For years, Dr. Herbert Benson from Harvard Medical School has studied Buddhist monks who practice a technique called G Tum-mo meditation.

Dr. Benson has repeatedly performed an experiment in which the monks are seated in a forty-degree room. Three-by-six-foot sheets are dipped in forty-nine-degree water and placed over the meditating monks' shoulders.

As Dr. Benson said, "For most people, such conditions would cause them to go into uncontrollable shivering and even death."

But it was not long before steam started rising from the monks' backs. And in approximately one hour, the sheets dried. Some monks are able to raise the temperatures of their fingers and toes by as much as seventeen degrees.

In another study, "Monks spent a winter night on a rocky ledge 15,000 feet high in the Himalayas. The sleep-out took place in February on the night of the winter full moon when temperatures reached zero degrees F. Wearing only woolen or cotton shawls, the monks promptly fell asleep on the rocky ledge. They did not huddle together, and the video shows no evidence of shivering. They slept until dawn then walked back to their monastery."

How is this possible?

The monks use a technique called "vase breathing" or abdominal breathing. Imagine that your abdomen is a vase, and every inhale fills the vase with fresh, clean water, starting with the bottom of your abdomen and all the way up to your collarbones. On the exhale, allow your abdomen to relax back as you pour the imaginary water out of the vase.

Researchers say this type of breathing causes thermogenesis which is a process of heat production. The monks also visualize that their breath is filled with fire moving up and down along their spine. The techniques, together, have an extraordinary effect.

These monks are not superhuman. They do not have a rare condition like synesthesia. They have spent years in deep meditation uncovering aspects of the brain that for most, lie frozen in the tundra of our subconscious.

## MEDITATE AND CELEBRATE

Make like The Magic Monks and take ten deep breaths to unleash the power of the mind.

According to many ancient Eastern traditions, breath is supremely powerful. In many languages the word for "breath" and the word for "spirit" are the same.

So why is it so rare that we utilize our breath?

In a twenty-four-hour period, we take approximately 20,000 breaths. Think about how many days go by where we don't even pay attention to a single breath.

I once saw Dr. Andrew Weil give a speech in which he said the single greatest health advice he can offer is to take ten deep breaths when you wake up in the morning, and ten deep breaths before you go to sleep at night.

Dr. Weil says, "Practicing regular, mindful breathing can be calming and energizing and can even help with stress-related health problems ranging from panic attacks to digestive disorders."

Has it been too long since you have stopped, and really enjoyed a good, long, deep, sweet inhale (and exhale)?

Conscious breathing is the first and best step to calming the mind and preparing for the magic to come.

**When you sit down to meditate, or go for a run, or need some extra power, try these words:**

*With the inhale, I am strong. With the exhale, I am free.*

*With the inhale, I am strong. With the exhale, I am free.*

*With the inhale, I am strong. With the exhale, I am free.*

# 27
## HURRY UP AND SLOW DOWN

---

### WHEN YOU EAT FAST, EVERYTHING IS FAST FOOD

In some way, you must be feeling the grind of life.

The grind is not just from an annoying coworker, screaming kids, or a flooding email inbox. There is a deeper reason behind the inherent human struggle that we all face every day: the Earth is an intensely foreign environment to the soul.

To function on Earth, the soul needs a spacesuit of sorts that we call skin, which is an absolute technological marvel.

As Diane Ackerman writes, "Our skin imprisons us, but it also gives us individual shape, protects us from invaders, cools us down or heats us up as need be and holds in our body fluids. Most amazing is that it can mend itself when necessary, and is constantly renewing itself. Skin can take a startling variety of shapes. It's waterproof, washable, and elastic."

So here we all are, souls in spacesuits, wandering Earth. And all this gravity, and "time," can make your soul loopy, similar to how elevation affects your brain. The loopiness creates static in our connection to Mission Control, which we call God, or the Universe, or an intelligence greater than our own. That's why we meditate or pray; it's a necessary step to connect with Mission Control.

But sometimes we forget to connect, to seek guidance, and we turn into a lost satellite, spinning our wheels until we burn out in the cold light of a distant sun. Ever feel that way?

It is an odd feeling, a shrill sensation that can be experienced any moment, regardless of your mood or physical surroundings.

In August 2012, I stood in Times Square with a huge crowd to watch NASA's Curiosity Mars rover land on the distant planet. It was a quintessential New York moment as I was shoulder to shoulder with hundreds of people from all over the world, watching this landmark achievement on giant, glittering screens.

But once it landed, there was nothing much to see. I wanted more.

The next morning, the headline read:

"After Trip of 352 Million Miles, Cheers for 23 Feet on Mars."

NASA sent the Mars rover initial instructions to roam only a short distance, testing out its connections and capabilities before sending it on further missions. It was not long before the rover was exploring hundreds of feet at a time, sending back brilliant images of the red rocks and ancient canyons on the Martian surface. But it all started with twenty-three feet.

We go through life feeling like we have done so much, traveled so far, yet we are barely moving forward.

I chose a very different path with a very different career trajectory. In some ways, I have the life experience of an 80 year old and in others, I feel like a 20 year old, as if I am just getting started.

Anais Nin wrote, "We do not grow absolutely, chronologically. We grow sometimes in one dimension, and not in another; unevenly. We grow partially. We are relative. We are mature in one realm, childish in another. The past, present, and future mingle and pull us backward, forward, or fix us in the present."

Slowly but surely, day by day, month by month, year by year, I have learned:

Stick with it! Keep going. And do not rush.

Mission Control will send you the signal, the moment, the person, the fortune you need to fulfill your mission. But first, you will be tested . . . sometimes only twenty-three feet at a time.

## MEDITATE AND CELEBRATE

Hurry up and slow down.

Nature is our greatest teacher and nature moves slowly.

Is it taking you way too long to fall in love?

Is growing your nest egg a painfully slow process?

Has your house been on the market for-freakin'-ever?

We all have something that is not happening fast enough.

Our culture places such an emphasis on speed, efficiency, and convenience. When you apply speed, efficiency, and convenience to things like your relationships or your evolution, it can be very unhealthy.

Try saying to your partner, "You know, we should hurry everything up. I'm in a rush to fall in love!" See how that goes over.

When you hear a child say "I just wanna grow up faster," you know it is the sparkle (and ignorance) of youth.

And if you saw someone trying to pry open the bud of a flower because the person did not have time to wait for it to bloom, would you not be dismayed that this wacko was ruining a perfectly beautiful flower?

So it goes when we rush our lives.

For many years, I have taught Yoga for Foodies workshops. While I am leading a yoga class, a chef is often right there in the room cooking up a feast. The participants can smell the aromas, hear the sizzle of the sauté pan, practically taste the flavors before they touch the palate.

It's about slowing down before tasting the subtleties of a deliciously prepared meal. The depth and nuances of the chef's work are lost if their creation is scarfed down. When we eat fast, everything might as well be fast food.

Speaking of fast food . . .

In 1986, McDonald's wanted to open near the Spanish Steps in Rome. After great protest, this triggered a movement to counter fast food with something called Slow Food, which promotes local foods and centuries-old traditions. Slow Food founder Carlos Petrini said, "Some things in life which are crucial to our maturity cannot be sped up, and are only possible if they occur slowly."

If you feel like you have done all the work, paid your dues, been patient, traveled 352 million miles with only twenty-three feet to show for it, take a deep breath and, as Emerson said, "adopt the pace of nature."

**On those days when you feel as if you will never get past those "twenty-three feet," soothe your impatience. Let these words help you take it down a notch:**

*Slow soothes, slow softens, slow heals.*

*Slow soothes, slow softens, slow heals.*

*Slow soothes, slow softens, slow heals.*

# 28
## STYLE YOUR THOUGHTS

**"I WILL NOT LET ANYONE
WALK THEIR DIRTY FEET
THROUGH MY MIND."
Gandhi**

I have never been one for fashion and style. I will be the first to tell you that there are insects that have better style. For instance, the butterfly has those fancy wings.

I wonder if a meager fly thinks, "There's that gosh darn butterfly with its fancy wings." In which case I would advise the meager fly, "Style is so much more than how you look."

What good is a mean person dressed in beautiful clothing? I would take a poorly dressed sweetheart any day of the week!

What is the point of a having great shoes if you are full of angry thoughts? I would rather live and die with a blissed out ragamuffin than a bitch of a fashionista.

Elizabeth Gilbert said, "You need to learn

how to select your thoughts just the same way you select your clothes every day."

So beware of what you are putting out there. Negative thoughts are bad style, let alone bad etiquette.

1. When you are entangled in an angry thought about an ex-lover, think of yourself in a tie-dye denim half shirt and knee pads. Angry thoughts are that ugly.
2. When you are dropping thought bombs on people that annoy you, think of yourself as a man in a pink g-string with a leather umbrella blocking the view of belligerent Buffalo Bills fans. Thought bombs are that bad.
3. When you are energy-slashing people with thought-sabres, think of yourself in a crotch-searing magenta unitard jogging down the Champs Elysses. Thought-sabres are extremely poor taste.

Be stylish, be classy, be beautiful, if not in what you wear, then certainly in how you think.

### MEDITATE AND CELEBRATE
Style your thoughts.

Start now by thinking three amazing thoughts. I'm talkin' funky, fancy, outrageous, gorgeous, powerful thoughts that define your truth and let your spirit exhale.

For example, here are three thoughts I love to ponder that make me feel happier, healthier, and "stylish."

## 1. "The Force Is Real"

Do you recall the very first *Star Wars* from the late 1970's? In the last scene, Jedi Master Luke Skywalker is attempting to destroy the Death Star. In this sci-fi world, Luke should use some futuristic device to get the job done. But no. The advice from his Jedi Master Obi-Wan Kenobi is "use your feelings Luke."

In a greatly symbolic moment, Luke switches off his high tech gadgets and taps into something greater than technology.

The Star Wars stories are largely inspired by philosopher Joseph Campbell's book *The Hero with a Thousand Faces.* Campbell worked closely with *Star Wars* creator George Lucas to fashion the Jedi Masters like those schooled in the ancient Eastern spiritual arts which emphasize mental prowess over physical prowess. Thus, the Jedi Masters embraced a deeper energy that binds everyone and everything. This energy is famously referred to as the Force.

How do you tap into the Force?

Every time you trust your intuition, it gets stronger.

Every time you follow your heart, it gets bolder.

Every time you lean on an Intelligence greater than your own, it draws closer.

You may never be able to move physical objects with your mind. But dabble with the Force and you will move people with your heart.

## 2. "Tension Rocks!"

A guitar, like any string instrument, is based on tension. If the strings are too loose or too tight, there can be no music.

So it goes with life. We all have tension. How you come to that tension says much about your sense of peace and harmony.

If your screaming kids are making you crazy, remember that one day your kids will grow up and move out. While the noise is there, let it remind you of the energy and vitality of youth. Today, can you be more patient with the noise and chaos at home?

If your house is a mess, so were the work desks of Mark Twain, Albert Einstein, and Steve Jobs. Hey, genius and creativity are messy processes. The 2nd Law of Thermodynamics states that everything in nature moves from order to disorder. The idea of being organized goes against the grain of the Universe. Can you come to "the mess" differently?

If you are mad at your partner, know that you would not be mad if you did not care. With great love comes great anger. It happens. Can you come to "mad" differently?

Take a moment and feel the particular way you are being pulled, challenged, and tried. What is making you tense? You have a choice: to bang "the guitar" to the ground in frustration or to strike your fingers to the chords and make music.

As Emerson wrote, "The world is all gates, all opportunities, all strings of tension waiting to be struck."

### 3. "Why Drive When You Can Fly?"

Imagine you are in the year 1769. You are living in a settlement in the newly formed territory of Pennsylvania. You wake up in your thatched hut to discover out front, an F-16 fighter jet. Being that it is 1769, you have no clue what you are looking at. Over time, you realize that you can climb into the F-16's cockpit. You play with the buttons and levers and realize this crazy thing can "propel" you forward on the ground. Years go by. You drive this F-16 fighter jet around a limited area. You are the talk of the territory. People come from near and far to marvel at this heap of mystery.

One night, while feeling a little crazy, you get into the jet and are driving so fast that you pull the lever and fly into the air! It is an accident, and you do not stay up for long.

But you actually fly!

Most of us, in some way, resemble the pilgrim with the F-16. We are toiling in our use of the complex machine known as the human brain. We are barely able to "drive," let alone take the great leap forward and fly.

It is time to evolve from the "driving stage" to the "flying stage" of our evolution. To evolve, we have to climb into the cockpit and take control.

From self-regulating our body temperature to performing instantaneous and complex calculations by calling upon our hidden synesthetic abilities, humans will be eventually be doing things with our minds that would seem like utter magic in today's world.

**When you are ready to make the shift from driving to flying, let your mind be your pilot, Jedi Master, and stylist. Repeat:**

*Powerful thoughts, powerful life.*

*Healthy thoughts, healthy life.*
*Loving thoughts, loving life.*

*Powerful thoughts, powerful life.*
*Healthy thoughts, healthy life.*
*Loving thoughts, loving life.*

*Powerful thoughts, powerful life.*
*Healthy thoughts, healthy life.*
*Loving thoughts, loving life.*

# 29
## PUT THE KIBOSH ON YOUR INNER CRITIC

---

**POWER IS A STATE OF AWARENESS**
We all have various people living within us, most of whom merit their own names.

For instance, within me there resides:

"Yeah Dave" who likes to hear himself talk, and ask questions just to be heard.

"Daaaaybeeeeed" who is similar to Warren from the movie *There's Something about Mary* and tends to get lost in confined spaces.

"Daveed" who is intellectual and loves to read Choose Your Own Adventure stories on fast trains.

"Romer" who tips the scale with Mexican Coca-Cola and late-night slices from South Brooklyn Pizza.

"Spaz" who chases tornadoes in his mind. "The sky is falling, the sky is falling!"

"D" who is relaxed, in the flow — my Highest Self. He can make you smile, laugh, and see all that is good and all that is right.

And then there is "Donald." Donald is my inner critic. He is a downer. He is the kind of guy who asks for peanut butter & jelly at a high-end Italian restaurant.

From awesome, loving, and generous to crazy, weird, and dubious, your various personalities may need to be enticed, but they are all there. I say, let them all live, let them all breathe, but do not let them all lead. Only your Highest Self should be President of your life.

So why do we continue to allow the insecure fool, the moody downer, the fear-driven freak to maintain control? It is hard to ward off the inner critic!

Let me tell you more about Donald. He says things like, "Brother Dave, you have manboobs, dude. Put down that slice of pizza. C'mon. There you go. Put. It. Down."

"Dave, gluten free is for sissies!"

"Dave, do you know what rhymes with 'hairy' and 'white?' YOUR LEGS! No shorts today. Or at least not those high riding shorts. Who are you?! John Stockton on the 1984 Utah Jazz? Disgusting bro!"

Here's the scary part. There were a good ten years when Donald was President of my life. He was the most vocal part of my mind, and he talked his way into power.

Maybe you can relate? Do you let the

unhealthy thoughts, made-up stories, anger, and resentment play a leading role in your daily existence?

There comes a time when you realize, "I don't have to and more importantly, I don't want to live like this."

## MEDITATE AND CELEBRATE

The inner critic will never go away, but there is a part of you who is far more qualified to lead. So put the kibosh on your inner critic. It is time for a coup! Take a moment to name your Highest Self and anoint Him/Her as President of your life.

One of my readers, Debbie, described her personal coup d'etat, "I realized letting go meant not of pain or tension but the weight of the inner critic I carried with me. I started to lighten up. I found myself more creative, loving, and spontaneous, noticing beautiful, funny, and delicious moments, sharing them with others and encouraging kids I work with to do the same. It was a small shift with a profound effect, a new flow that cost me absolutely nothing and added so much value to my life."

Debbie is describing the most powerful action you can take when facing the inner critic. Appreciation. Whether it's being more loving to yourself or saying the words you never take the time to say to the person you never take the time to love, appreciation is the finest quality of your Highest Self. It is realizing you already have what you need to rise to power. Author Shakti Gawain wrote, "To think you need something you don't already have is a form of insanity."

And if you want to really put the figure-four leglock on your inner critic, here is the secret. Luxuriate. Your Higher Self wants to be treated like royalty and enjoy what Debbie calls "the beautiful, funny, and delicious moments" in the day. Take the extra few minutes to lie in bed before you wake up. Go for the $10 foot massage. Treat yourself to the best piece of chocolate you have ever tasted.

Luxuriate.

Appreciate.

**And repeat the words that can only be spoken by your Highest Self:**

*When the chocolate flows,*
*My power grows.*

*When the chocolate flows,*
*My power grows.*

*When the chocolate flows,*
*My power grows.*

# 30
## Sleep Like a Four-Year-Old

### If Sleep Is a Sport, Let Me Be Champion

He is my wife's "boyfriend."

He is more handsome than me.

He has a better physique.

He brings her great pleasure.

He takes her to the most exotic places.

He treats her to the finest meals in the greatest restaurants. He knows secrets about her that I do not.

He seems to say all the right things.

Does "he" make me jealous? HELL YEAH! How can I possibly withstand this relationship? It gets worse.

She spends eight hours per day, fifty-six hours per week, 240 hours per month, and 2,920 hours per year with this "boyfriend."

Before you jump to conclusions, let me explain.

These are the thoughts that run through my head while I watch my wife sleep deeply.

I will spend nights tossing and turning, just staring at her with her shit-eating sleepy-time grin. Such is her bedtime bliss that it appears each night as if she is having a rendezvous with a boyfriend . . . in her dreams. In truth, this boyfriend is sleep itself.

To my fellow insomniacs, I say to you, "Oh, the things we think about at 3:42 AM on sleepless nights."

Maybe one out of seven nights I sleep well, but the rest of the time, I will skim the surface of consciousness. I am awakened by the slightest movement, like an ant roaming across the floor. And in a big city with lots of noise right outside my window, I hope for moments, rather than complete hours of sleep.

With all the caffeine, frightening news, and intense stress that most adults sustain, it is tough for the adult brain to completely shut down for eight hours at a time.

I actually think sleep was designed for children. And that is the trick to sleeping better at night. If you would not read it or show it to your four-year-old before going to sleep, it will probably keep you up at night.

For instance:

—Would you ever read your four-year-old a bedtime story about a despotic leader amassing arms to destroy the world while his citizens starve to death? Then why would you read the latest magazine article about some dictator on the other side of the planet?

—Would you ever show your four-year-old a scary movie about a plane crashing just before bedtime? Of course not! So why on a recent Friday night did I watch a movie about a plane crash just as I was brushing my teeth and getting ready for bed?

—Would you ever let your four-year-old sip a third glass of wine? As much as you might enjoy a cocktail, many people have a hard time sleeping properly after consuming alcohol.

I know, I know, I know. You are not a four-year-old. But if you are one of the 48 percent of Americans who report occasional insomnia or one of the 22 percent who endure insomnia every single night, might it be time for a new approach?

## MEDITATE AND CELEBRATE
Sleep like a baby by catering to your inner four-year-old in the minutes before bedtime.

— Read something relaxing, joyful, pleasant, and funny at the end of your day. It is a gift to your mind to fade out peacefully.

— Wear super comfy clothes (aka PJs). I will never forget that time when I was six, and my dad told me the confining consequences of wearing tighty-whities to bed at night. Never again.

— Share five things for which you are grateful. It really helps to end the day with a note of positivity. As Dr. Robert Emmons said, "If you want to sleep more soundly, count blessings, not sheep."

— Turn down the lights. No blinking screens while lying in bed. Let the mind wind down rather than rev up. *The New York Times* reported, "Researchers at Rensselaer Polytechnic Institute showed that exposure to light from computer tablets significantly lowered levels of the hormone melatonin, which regulates our internal clocks and plays a role in the sleep cycle."

Consider putting as much emphasis on getting ready for bed as you would on getting ready for your day. Slow things down, relax your mind, and surround yourself with the right reading, soothing lighting, relaxing smells, and a sweet surrender into a dream-time adventure.

If you need a little lullaby when you are tossing and turning on a sleepless night, these are the words of the late, great yogi Larry Schultz (who happened to be private yoga teacher to the Grateful Dead). They are as relevant to a good sleeper as they are to a relaxed yogi:

*Nowhere to go. No one to be. Nothing to do.*

*Nowhere to go. No one to be. Nothing to do.*

*Nowhere to go. No one to be. Nothing to do.*

# 31
## BE THE MIRACLE

**NOW IS ALWAYS THE BEST MOMENT**
While having a very disappointing phone conversation, I walked by a despondent homeless man, his hat in his hand, hoping for change.

I had a big bag of spare change in my briefcase that I saved up to donate to the right person. I dropped it in the homeless man's hat.

This homeless man expected pennies, maybe quarters, one or two at a time.

But my bag of change must have weighed three pounds, and the man was shocked when his hat almost fell out of his hand.

He instantly lit up. Life returned to his face.

And the effect that once-disappointing call had on my psyche instantly dissipated, thanks to my helper's high, a scientifically proven dopamine-mediated euphoria resulting from an altruistic action. Hey, everyone loves a buzz, and the natural ones are the best kind!

To the homeless man, this was a minor miracle. To me, this was a major revelation.

In the midst of my despondent phone call in which I was waiting to hear about a potential opportunity, I realized how much time I spend waiting. Waiting to make more money, waiting to launch my new business, waiting to be the recipient of a big shot's good graces.

Enough with the waiting! YOU ARE THE BIG SHOT.

You Are The Miracle.

As philosopher David Hawkins said, "There's nothing out there other than consciousness itself."

What's in here is out there. Nothing is gonna happen to you that does not first happen within you. If you want a miracle, be the miracle. Go create one. NOW. Give money, give medicine, give love.

And here is an idea for a super sweet gift that does not cost you a dime:

WISDOM!

To receive another's wisdom is like tasting years of hard-earned life lessons distilled into one sweet drop. And when that wisdom falls unexpectedly into your lap and presents a wormhole to another perspective, a new frequency, a revitalized energy, now that is a miracle!

Whether it is giving advice to someone just starting out on a similar career path, or consoling someone with a broken heart, your everyday wisdom might just be another's breakthrough.

## MEDITATE AND CELEBRATE

Be the miracle and share your hard-earned wisdom.

Here is a little exercise to stir up all the juicy wisdom in your soul. Write your own commencement address.

To inspire you, let's look back at these great moments in the history of commencement addresses (including my own):

### Bono to the University of Pennsylvania in 2004

"I love America because America is not just a country, it's an idea. You see my country, Ireland, is a great country, but it's not an idea. America is an idea, but it's an idea that brings with it some baggage, like power brings responsibility. It's an idea that brings with it equality, but equality, even though it's the highest calling, is the hardest to reach. The idea that anything is possible, that's one of the reasons why I'm a fan of

America. It's like 'Hey, look there's the moon up there, let's take a walk on it, bring back a piece of it.' That's the kind of America that I'm a fan of."

### Steve Jobs to Stanford in 2005

"Death is very likely the single best invention of life. It's life's change agent; it clears out the old to make way for the new . . . Your time is limited so don't waste it living someone else's life. Don't be trapped by dogma, which is living with the results of other people's thinking. Don't let the noise of others' opinions drown out your own inner voice, heart and intuition."

### Nora Ephron to her alma mater Wellesley in 1996

"Whatever you choose, however many roads you travel, I hope that you choose not to be a lady. I hope you will find some way to break the rules and make a little trouble out there. And I also hope that you will choose to make some of that trouble on behalf of women."

### Brian Williams, George Washington University in 2012

"You don't actually have to build a rocket or go into space, but please take us somewhere. Please keep us moving. Push us, lift us up. Make us better."

## Sheryl Sandberg to Barnard College in 2011

"Don't let your fears overwhelm your desire. Let the barriers you face — and there will be barriers — be external, not internal. Fortune does favor the bold, and I promise that you will never know what you're capable of unless you try."

## Dave Romanelli to some graduation class in the Future

There are many ways to miss life. Stressed for time. Anxious for money. Drowning in minutiae.

There are many ways to enjoy life. Taking it easy. Pushing your limits. Following your passion.

There are many ways to taste life. Sweet, sour, salty.

There is only one way and one word to CELEBRATE life. That word is NOW.

Never wait to celebrate.

The older you get, the more you will realize that people don't change. Someone who was a worrier in his twenties is still worrying in his forties. Someone who was regretful in her forties is still that way in her eighties. The only way to break the pattern is this:

Never wait to celebrate.

The present is ALWAYS the best moment. Not because it is the happiest moment, but because it is the moment you are most alive. If yesterdays and tomorrows come at the cost of todays, you have forgotten these words:

Never wait to celebrate.

When I lived in New York City and was getting worn down by the pace, someone gave me this advice, which is true not just about New York City but about something much greater. "Life will take a lot from you, so you take a lot from life." You know the words.

NEVER WAIT TO CELEBRATE.

The one who honors the simple pleasures and small victories wins the game of life over and over again.

NEVER WAIT TO CELEBRATE.

As seen in a 111-year-old woman in NYC whose tips for living fully are not play it safe but rather sex, vodka, and spicy food . . .

NEVER WAIT TO CELEBRATE.

As advised by a young woman lost before her fortieth birthday, "What I would give for another year. In my memory, celebrate another year every day!"

NEVER WAIT TO CELEBRATE.

How do you put this theory into practice?
There is only way and one word.

NOW!